Learning from Patients:

My Life as a Student Nurse

John R. Blakeman, RN

ISBN 13: 978-1-5076-3685-5

*To my family, friends, and professors who
have made this journey possible and especially to my Grandpa,
Robert "Bob" Gaither, who had a tremendous impact on my
life and influenced me to choose nursing . . .*

I yelled to my partner to "tell them he is not breathing and has no pulse – CPR in progress." I knew I had a bag-valve mask in my medical bag (one of the tools that are commonly seen in television shows and movies when medical personnel are "bagging" a patient – squeezing a football-looking bag that is delivering air to the patient), and I knew that the patient's wife was on oxygen at night and had a portable oxygen tank.

I ran to grab the portable tank and also my bag valve mask and very quickly hooked up the bag to the oxygen. This took maybe 20 seconds, as I was in turbo mode. By that time, my partner was back. "Here, you do airway and bag," I said, as I started compressions.

"One, two, three . . ." I counted rapidly as I compressed the patient's chest. I could feel a crack here and there – likely ribs cracking under the pressure of my compressions . . .

CONTENTS

PREFACE

Writing a "memoir" is a lot harder than it sounds. I could not believe the amount of time it took – not to actually write this book (which did take quite a bit of time) but to wrap my mind around my entire experience in nursing school. With so much happening in the four years I was in school, it was no easy task figuring out what stories I wanted to share, what messages I wanted to send and how I wanted to organize it all.

While many of the stories that I tell in this book I could recall from memory because they made such a significant impact on me, I also utilized a journal that I kept during nursing school. I sometimes recorded my thoughts in writing, and I also made my own video logs, especially when I was busy and did not have time to stop and write my thoughts out. Also, each clinical day during nursing school required me to write a reflection, so I was able to reference those clinical reflections in writing this book as well. Of course, patient confidentiality has always taken top priority, and in the majority of cases, I cannot even remember patient names, as these are not included in my reflections.

I should note that the stories in this book have been edited to remove or change identifying details. Because confidentiality is so incredibly important, I have altered several details about patients. However, the major events and lessons learned from the patients have remained the same. Also, I have chosen not to identify the hospitals I worked in. My experience at each of the hospitals was different, and there were certainly pros and cons about each; however, I feel that there is no need to name specific hospitals in my discussion, as it is not an integral part of my stories. Further, I have not included every single patient story and all details of my time in nursing school, simply because this book would be 1,000 pages long if I did.

At any rate, I hope a wide variety of readers find things book interesting. While it is certainly applicable to nursing students, the many stories contained in this book reveal something interesting about society. The stories explicate the delicacy of human life and how many of us take for granted what we truly have.

INTRODUCTION

Coming to Nursing

It took me a while to decide to become a nurse. Quite honestly, I had not considered being a nurse until my junior year of high school, and it was not until my senior year that I made the definitive decision. I suppose it shouldn't have come as a surprise to me; after all, I was ecstatic to receive a toy IV kit for Christmas when I was in elementary school. Not many other children could claim that this item was at the top of their "best all-time Christmas gifts" list.

As a child, I wanted to be (in order) a firefighter, a police officer, a physician, a criminal intelligence analyst, a physician (again), a meteorologist, a teacher, and a nurse. Firefighter, police officer, doctor (the first time) and criminal intelligence analyst do not really count, though. When I have looked back at old preschool videos, it seemed that every child wanted to be a doctor, firefighter, or police officer. I suppose that these careers are highlighted in childrens' early lives, and so when asked what they want to be when they grow up, small children will typically give these careers as answers. As for criminal intelligence analyst, my aunt Anne turned me onto this career when I was in second or third grade. She worked for the Illinois State Police and had heard about this field through her job. She told me about it, and since I had such a love for my aunt, I of course instantly wanted to be a criminal intelligence analyst.

As I grew older, I realized how much I actually liked medicine, and, for the second time, I turned my attention to becoming a physician. Shows like ER had given me a basis for what a physician does, so I would "play doctor" frequently, forcing my stuffed animals to suffer through terrible attempts at administering an IV correctly (as correctly as an IV can be administered by an eight-year-old). Though I really wanted to become a physician, I did not limit myself to that role. I spent countless hours playing paramedic in my mother's van, folding down the seats (or removing them fully) so that I could fit the usual yellow plastic snow sled in the back. Typically, I would pretend some catastrophic event had occurred and then would "respond" to the scene in my "rescue truck," which was typically a pedal car with wagon attached. Upon arrival, I would immobilize the victim, usually a stuffed dog or bear, by putting toilet paper rolls or wash cloths on either side of the "patient's" head. After that, I would start IVs and cover any serious "wounds" with band aids. If you ask any of my former neighbors about it, they would verify the information, as I know they saw me in the front or back yard tending to my patients. After I loaded them onto the yellow sled, I would urgently place them in the back of the van and hop in with them, giving shots and taking their blood pressure while the "ambulance" was en route to the hospital. Once the ambulance arrived at the hospital, I would jump out and become the emergency physician, ordering x-rays and asking for labs. This routine continued for a few years until I turned my attention to meteorology.

For about two years from 5th grade to 6th grade, I wanted to be your weather man. In fact, I wrote an essay about wanting to be a meteorologist and ended up delivering the morning weather for a local television station after being a winner in their essay contest. I am not quite sure what was so appealing about becoming a meteorologist. I guess it was probably the fact that I was intrigued with the formation of storms and how so much energy could be used and released by nature.

After meteorology, teaching popped onto the radar. My mom and several grandparents had all been teachers, and so I was very familiar with the field. Though I knew this career choice would not come with much pay, I loved the idea of teaching people (and still do). Being able to convey information to others has always interested me, and so teaching seemed like the perfect profession for me. In fact, I wanted to be a teacher from about 7th grade until the end of my junior year of high school.

In May 2008, however, my grandpa was hospitalized with a severe infection in his digestive tract. All-in-all he was in the hospital for 9 days and underwent countless blood tests and medication adjustments. While this was an unhappy time in my grandfather's life, it was positively life-changing for me. For three nights, my grandpa had the same nurse, Beth Young. Beth was an excellent nurse that treated my grandpa well and also kept us (the family) informed. She even called early one morning to give us the update after they had made a significant medication change.

On Beth's last night as my grandpa's nurse, she told me, "You would be a great nurse. Have you ever thought about nursing?"

I responded truthfully by saying "no" that I had not ever thought about nursing.

Beth then told me of the many benefits of nursing and encouraged me to investigate the profession further. A few weeks after my conversation with Beth, I was talking with Andy Goodall, a firefighter-paramedic from my hometown of Taylorville, Illinois. He reinforced Beth's words by encouraging me to look at nursing since so many opportunities exist for males in the nursing profession.

Not only did I want to be able to help people and provide great care like Beth, but also, I looked at more and more statistics and realized just how many options and avenues are available to nurses. I began to change my mind from teaching to nursing. However, my decision to choose nursing over teaching was not so much a choice of one over another but rather a choice of both. Nursing allows not only teaching patients about their illnesses, medications, and so forth, but it also allows individuals to become nurse educators, serving in various settings including in hospitals and colleges. I will be able to fulfill many of my life desires such as helping people and solving difficult medical issues but also enrich others' lives through teaching by being a nurse educator some day.

Once I decided upon nursing, I had to find a college, and I knew I wanted to earn my bachelor of science in nursing, also sometimes referred to as the "four year nursing degree," since it requires four years to complete. There are also associate degree nursing programs which tend to require around three years total of schooling, and very few "diploma programs," though these are few and far between across the nation. Diploma programs have no degree tied to them – only the ability to sit for the national licensing exam, the NCLEX. In a lot of practice settings, nurses with a bachelor's degree have a higher pay scale, and some studies have suggested that the more education a nurse has, the better patient outcomes tend to be.

After browsing through information about several colleges, I decided upon Millikin University in Decatur, Illinois, because it was small enough that I could be engaged with faculty members and wouldn't be "just another number." The school also had a very high pass rate on the nursing licensing exam and was not too far from home. I was able to apply early and was accepted in the fall of my senior year of high school.

My four years at Millikin would be challenging yet rewarding, energizing yet tiring, but, most of all, they were worthwhile. Many people have asked me if I knew what I do now, would I have chosen to pursue a degree in nursing, and my answer is always a resounding "yes." It was not easy, but it was most definitely a life-changing experience.

PART I: WELCOME TO NURSING

Ch. 1:
Welcome to Nursing School

As I guided my trusty, harvest gold Ford Ranger into the parking space next to the tall nursing and science building at my university, I scanned the parking lot, noticing a few other students that looked to be about my age slowly meandering towards the door, tall coffee cups in hand, undoubtedly containing some extra-strength java. Nobody looked too awake; it was before 8:00 AM, after all, and it was still technically winter break, so none of us were in the mood to be back on campus.

It was quite a shock when we received a letter in the mail three weeks prior informing us that we would need to come back to campus several days early in order to attend nursing orientation. Many of us asked (some rather furiously) the same question: "How can they expect us to be at school when the semester hasn't even started?"

Of course, as the semesters went on, we all learned that in nursing school and nursing in general, nothing is off limits – not even reading assignments that come a few weeks before the start of the semester or review sessions on weekends. We would also begin to appreciate that this sort of "all in" attitude is of value in the nursing school and the nursing profession.

As I made my way into the deserted-looking building, I saw some golden light shining into the hallway from a room down the hall – room 112, which would become well known to all of us, since we would spend countless hours there listening to lectures, studying and practicing various skills on each other and the rather mysterious looking manikins in the back of the classroom. These manikins somehow changed from males to females and back again, depending on which toupées were placed on their heads and which genitalia were attached. Each of these plastic humanoids went from Mr. Smith one day to Mrs. Hernandez the next. What a confusing life they lead.

I turned the corner into the room, and there were already six or eight students sitting at the long desks, with a combination of tiredness, fear and stress on their faces. As I sat down, Ian, a fellow male nursing student (We would eventually term ourselves the "murses.") said hello and asked how my winter break had been. I'm sure my answer was something along the lines of "It wasn't nearly long enough…" While the others had the look of desperation on their faces, I'm sure I had the same look on my face.

Since the program I was enrolled in was a four year, Bachelor of Science in Nursing program, we had already spent a year and a half together in foundational classes, such as microbiology, anatomy and physiology, public speaking, organic/biochemistry, psychology, and the list goes on. It was now time to begin our nursing classes where we would learn how to care for patients and what certain diseases were and how they should be treated. We would also take part in infamous "clinicals."

I know I was terrified to begin the "real" part of nursing school. Up to this point, none of us had really taken a true nursing course. But now, we would begin our courses in basic nursing skills, health assessment, pharmacology, pathophysiology, research and management, mental health nursing, maternal/child nursing, medical-surgical nursing and community health nursing.

Perhaps the most daunting part of our "real" nursing classes was clinicals. Our clinicals essentially entailed going to a practice setting (hospital, outpatient clinic, house, etc.) and doing what a nurse does, on top of all of our other classes. Though every nursing school is different, clinicals usually involve one instructor with somewhere between six and twelve students. Each student is generally assigned one to two patients and is responsible for that patient – passing medications, providing therapeutic communication, starting IVs, inserting Foley catheters into urinary bladders . . . you name it, really. Clinicals also involve hours upon hours of paperwork, before and after. In my case, clinicals were almost always on Tuesday and Thursday, which meant I had to gather patient information at the hospital the night before (though some clinicals were slightly different). For every day of clinical, I would spend approximately six to ten hours on paperwork for that one day of clinical – twelve to twenty hours for the entire week. That didn't include the many hours of studying for my other classes, sleep, meetings, engagements involving student organizations, and a "social life" (which seemed rather non-existent at times). It's easy to see how the start of clinical rotations was a bit intimidating for all of us. We knew what was coming, and we knew we weren't going to like it. Though as the days went on, I think we all learned a lot about ourselves and about humanity as a whole, and, though it might seem a bit touchy-feely, clinicals made it all worth it.

Even though we had spent three semesters together already, we really didn't know one another that well because we hadn't *needed* to know each other that well yet. Yes, we knew one another's names, and we knew some minor details about each other, depending on what cliques we had been a part of for the prior year and a half. But we didn't *know* each other.

I make such a big deal about getting to know each other because, by the end of nursing school, we all *did* know each other. We were (and still are, in many cases) a family by the time we finished the 5 long semesters of our nursing courses. We knew intimate details about each others' lives, and we could tell when something was off with a classmate. When a member of the family was down and out, the rest of the class would try to pick him or her up. It's no wonder that we became so close, either. Nursing school basically forces students to work together and to form support groups, not only for studying and figuring out the best study strategies but also for the 2:00 AM phone calls or 5:00 AM text messages that, during times of extreme stress, are highly needed. We all needed a shoulder to cry on or an ear to vent to at times, and I don't think that there is a single nursing student in my class that did not think about quitting nursing school, at least once. But it's the family atmosphere and support from one another that got us through.

More and more students shuffled in to the rather stuffy classroom, and we even noted some new faces that we had never seen before. These people were transfer students, and they fit right in with the rest of us – scared, tired and unsure of the future.

Right at 8:00 AM, two of our professors walked in and welcomed us. It was then time for introductions, and we went around the room stating our name, where we were from, what area of nursing we were interested in and one interesting fact about ourselves. As a side note, I have always been annoyed by that last question. It's hard to come up with something interesting. How does one state something that is interesting without sounding like a braggart but also come up with something that is truly, well, interesting. At any rate, we made it through.

I stated that I was interested in geriatrics and got the "Why?" look from just about everyone in the class. (Since that day, I've gotten the same look time after time when I tell people that I really enjoy working with older adults.) The majority of the students seemed to want to do something related to children or mothers – pediatrics, obstetrics or neonatal nursing. I was certainly the odd person out wanting to work with older adults.

After the formalities, we were handed a syllabus for our introductory nursing course and another health assessment course. After flipping through some of the pages, the stress level in the room skyrocketed. In a matter of a day, we had all gone from blissful winter break relaxation to full panic mode. We all saw how many assignments we had for the semester, and we also noted that we had a fairly lengthy reading assignment for the following Monday, our first day of classes. There would undoubtedly be a quiz, we were certain. (As it turned out, there was no quiz, but we were ready for one, no doubt.) All of the assignments and expectations listed in the syllabi were very overwhelming. I don't think any of us knew how we would get it all done.

To make matters worse, we were aware that the grading scale for the school of nursing was much harder than any of us had ever experienced before. After all, a 77% was passing. Anything below that, even a 76.99%, was failing, and none of us could afford (in many cases literally) to fail.

We were guided through the school of nursing handbook after the syllabi. "No visible tattoos, only two stud-type earrings, polished shoes, pressed uniforms," and the list went on. Our uniforms were to consist of the school-issued navy scrub top and scrub pants finished with bright, all-white shoes. We were also issued a white lab coat. At that point, we all took this information quite seriously. Several of us ran out to buy clothing steamers, actually.

Finally, to wrap up the rather long and tedious morning, the director of the school of nursing, Dr. Ramirez, presented a short message. It was half warning and half pep talk.

"For some of you, nursing school will come more naturally," she said. "You will wake up for clinical one day and say, 'I feel like a nurse.' For others, it might take more time, but you will get there."

While she encouraged us and said that we could all do well and pass all of our classes, she also made sure we knew we would have to work our fannies off and that we would need to make some sacrifices in our lives.

"It's not easy. You will have to work hard and be ready to change what you know," she said.

I don't blame her for this warning, either, because she was right.

She also reminded us that nursing is a profession and is special. In Illinois, nurses aren't actually just "registered nurses" as most people call them. A nursing license actually lists an RN as a "registered *professional* nurse." A lot of people don't know this fact, and I didn't know it until Dr. Ramirez told us.

She emphasized that "You aren't just there to do tasks like start IVs and give medications. You are there to notice the subtle changes in patients, to provide support and comfort even in the final hours of patients' lives. What you do is special. You have made the decision to make a difference, and you will make a difference."

It was in that moment that I think we all remembered why we were doing what we were doing. After the morning of stress and worry, it was nice to be reminded why we wanted to be nurses.

Sure, some of my classmates were in it for the job security and good pay, but many of us chose nursing because we saw our passion in the profession. And even some of those that decided upon nursing for the more tangible reasons ended up finding their passion in nursing. I would wager to say that to graduate from nursing school, it takes passion. Without passion, there is no drive to get through the late nights and the early mornings and the stressful days in between.

As I walked out of classroom 112, my mind began to float to imagining what my first clinical day, just about five weeks away, would be like. How would I act? What would I say? Would I be able to make the patient and possibly the patient's family believe that I knew what I was doing? Would I even know what I was doing? As these questions raced through my mind, I set my sights on what was most important – surviving nursing school.

The various chapters of this book all point out different lessons that nursing school taught me. And it taught me a lot!

As those next five semesters trudged along, I learned. I learned about health care. I learned how to do nursing tasks like start IVs and change surgical dressings. I learned how to talk to suicidal patients. I learned so much that I can't remember what all I learned. But even more importantly, I learned about myself and about humanity. I learned what it means to be compassionate and empathetic.

I learned what it really means to be a nurse.

Ch. 2:
Zero Hour – Clinical, Day 1

The first several weeks of my introductory nursing course, Intro Practicum in Nursing, had gone by, and it was now time to put all that we had learned into practice.

We were taught how to give baths, empty catheters, take vital signs, make beds (with and without a patient in the bed) and do a host of other tasks, but would we actually be able to do all of these things in the clinical setting? I think we all wondered that throughout nursing school.

The night before, I had gone to the hospital to get my patient assignment. Our clinical instructor posted the assignments in the employee break room on the medical unit we were on, so my first task would be to go to that room to look up my assignment. I entered the main hallway of the unit and located the break room. Sitting there were two older nurses, talking about staffing for the next day. Of course, they were sitting right in front of the clinical assignment list, posted on the bulletin board.

"Great. I'm going to have to ask them to move, and they are going to tell me to get a life, since I'm a nursing student," I thought. "I'll be annoying them asking them to move."

I looked around for about a minute, not really doing anything, hoping that by some miracle they would decide to get up. No such luck. After taking a minute to twiddle my thumbs awkwardly, I inched toward them and asked them if I could sneak between them to look at my assignment for the next day.

To my surprise I received the response, "Of course! Will this be your first day of clinical?" from one of the two nurses sitting at the table.

What!? No snide comment? No frown or sarcastic remark? I had heard how mean and unwelcoming all of the nurses would be, but, so far, this picture was not coming true.

Even though it was such a minor encounter, those two nurses being nice to me made a world of difference. They gave me hope that clinical would not be as bad as I had imagined, and they taught me that I needed to go into everything I was going to do in nursing school with an open mind.

Indeed, that is one major piece of advice for nursing students. While it is important to learn from upperclassmen and find out what is important to know, what certain professors like to quiz about, and so forth, some things also have to be taken with a grain of salt. Have some of the upper classmen had bad experiences with staff nurses? Yes. However, that does not mean that every nursing student is going to have a bad experience. In nursing school, the majority of the time "it is what you make of it."

After this not-so-terrible encounter, I made my way to the nursing station so that I could log onto the computer to find out information about my patient. All I knew was that I had a 78-year-old male and what room he was in. I was relieved, though, that I would have a male. It was not that I was uncomfortable taking care of a female, but I was worried that a female patient might refuse to allow me to take care of her.

The computer worked the first time (not always the case), and I was able to log in to the charting system with no problems. I located the patient room and double clicked on the patient's name. Ahhhh. It was finally time to "meet" my first patient. The diagnosis read "bilateral shingles." At the time, I did not realize how unusual this was. We had not had pathophysiology up to that point, so many of the diseases' causes and progressions were unknown to us. However, shingles, a painful rash caused by the same herpes zoster virus that causes chicken pox, almost always only affects one side of the body (in approximately 96% of cases) – left or right. It follows nerve paths, or dermatomes, and does not normally cross the "midline," an imaginary line that runs vertically, splitting the body in half. However, in this patient's case, his shingles affected both sides of his body, indicating he was a fairly sick man. I collected all of the information I would need – things such as his diet, activity level, notable laboratory values and pretty much anything else that I might need to develop a care plan. I also wrote down all of his eighteen medications. I would have a long night ahead of me writing down all of these medications, their particular characteristics, side effects, normal dosage ranges and a lot of other important information.

Because I was not used to the computer system, it took me two hours to gather the necessary data. However, I got there eventually.

When I got back to my apartment, I plopped down on the couch in the living room next to one of my roommates with my stack of books, ready to look up the patient's medications and figure out what my priority nursing interventions would be. He was a little confused why I had been to the hospital already that night, since I would be going there the next day. But by that point, he was accustomed to the unusual things I did in regard to studying and preparation for class.

Three and a half hours later, I was done. I set my alarm for 5:30 AM and chose the most annoying ring tone I could find as my notification. And the next morning, right on schedule, my phone came to life with the most annoying whistling sound I have ever heard. Incidentally, I used this same ring tone throughout my time in nursing school – not because I liked it but because it was irritating enough to wake me up even when my body didn't want to be woken up. (When I purchased a new phone my senior year, I actually downloaded the specific ring tone so that I could continue my ring tone tradition. In retrospect, this action may have been a bit over-board, but it relieved my nerves at the time, so it was worth it.)

I rolled out of bed, having only gotten about three hours of sleep due to my anxiety the night before. I spent most of the night tossing and turning, picturing how horrible my first day of clinical would be. I just knew I would have the worst patient who would not want a student nurse, and I knew he or she would point out all of my mistakes to me.

As I stumbled across my room, searching for the light switch, I glanced over at my laptop computer, which I had just turned on before jumping out of bed. The text in the upper right hand corner of the screen showed the temperature, on this particular morning a chilly 10 degrees Fahrenheit. It was February in Illinois, so I guess I could have expected it to be that cold.

I made my way to the shower, thinking all the way, "It's as cold as a wrought iron toilet seat on the shady side of an iceberg." I tended to use that phrase when it was extremely cold outside, and many of my classmates got a good laugh the first time they heard me say it.

After taking my shower and fully waking myself up, it was time to put on my scrubs – excuse me, my uniform – for "real" for the first time. After putting on my pants and shirt, I went through the checklist of things I would need. Stethoscope? Check. Wrist watch? Check. Pens? Check. Pen light? Check. Note pad? Check. Bandage scissors? Check. Confidence? Uhhh. Not so much.

Glancing at my watch, I noticed that it was 6:15 AM. Ian would be picking me up in five minutes, so I slipped on my polished, all-white shoes, and made my way to the front of the apartment complex. He was already there when I got there, looking just about as nervous as me. We buzzed our way across town and made it to the hospital well before we had to be there. Clinical started at 7:00 AM, but most of us were there by 6:30, fearing that we might be late.

The day was honestly a blur. There were eight of us in this clinical group, and to start out the day, each of us gave a summary of the patients we had. Our professor asked us individual questions that we were expected to know the answer to, though most of the questions we answered as a team.

After finding out that bilateral shingles were so rare during my research the night before, I figured that might be a question I would be asked. And, in fact, she did ask me "What makes your patient's diagnosis so unusual?" I was happy that I was able to answer this first question correctly because I felt that I was starting this clinical off on the right foot. Surprisingly, that was the only question I was asked, most likely because we were already a little behind schedule.

My hours of clinical went fairly smoothly – well after I started out with a rather embarrassing blunder. When I was initially introducing myself, the patient asked me if I could help him reposition, which I happily agreed to. However, when I began to move the head of the bed down, I forgot to remove everything from under the upper part of the bed, and I ended up smashing the trash can under the bed. When the force on the can got too great, it made a loud "pop" and shot out from under the bed. Needless to say, I was embarrassed, and from that point forward I made sure I checked for hazards before I changed bed positions. No harm, no foul – I chalked it up to a learning experience. It was moments like these that I learned not to downplay or ignore. I realized pretty early on in nursing school how important it was to learn from my mistakes and to reflect on them. To this day, I find this attitude very valuable.

My patient was quite polite, and the family that was present in the room always smiled. This patient did not require much direct care at all, since he was independent. He shaved himself and gave himself a bath, and all I had to do was change his sheets. I also went through the usual assessment questions with him, finding out when his last bowel movement was and if he was having any pain.

I did his head-to-toe physical assessment, not necessarily even knowing what I was doing the entire time, since we had not totally completed our health assessment course at that point. He knew who he was, where he was, and what year it was, so he was alert and oriented times three (also known as A&O x 3). His heart sounded good, along with his lungs, and his bowels were moving normally – not that I had heard that many "normal" heart, lung and bowel sounds. Strength was good in his arms and legs, and his only problem seemed to be the extreme pain he was in.

At the end of our four hour day (clinicals during our first clinical rotation were shorter), I said goodbye to my patient and his family and packed up my things. We gave a quick report to the nurse that would be assuming care for our patients and headed for the exits.

I felt like I had given good care to my patient, but about a year and a half later, I realized that I did not get to know my patient as well as I should have. Interestingly, while flipping through the local paper, I came across a name.

"This name sounds so familiar, I thought. Why do I know this name?"

Then, it hit me. It was my first ever patient. He had passed away the day before. In reading his obituary, I found out that he had served for almost four decades in the military and had an assortment of medals and awards. He had invented several items and held patents on them. Further, he volunteered almost daily at a local homeless shelter, helping to provide services to some of the most vulnerable in the community.

I had known none of this prior to reading his obituary. I felt as though I had somehow let my patient down. When taking care of him, I asked essentially no questions about his life. I thought that I had been a tremendous communicator, and in my clinical reflection for the day, I even recorded,

> "I really was impressed by the way I communicated with family members in the room of my patient. When the patient's wife and granddaughter visited, I was able to continue to care for the patient while also engaging in conversation with the family members. This allowed me to be able to make the family members feel more relaxed with me caring for their loved one and also likely helped the patient feel better. I think that my ability to communicate was not limited to the family though; I also was successful at communicating with the patient. He seemed to respond well to me, and at the end of the day, he even shook my hand and thanked me for what I had done; this certainly made me feel good."

That day, I forgot to see what his home life was like. While I very superficially communicated with the patient, about things like the weather, the latest current events and the air temperature of the room, I didn't get to know the patient as an individual. What did he do in his spare time? I didn't know – until I read his darn obituary.

Of course, by the time I read his obituary, I had become better at therapeutic communication with patients, so I was, at that point, asking all of my patients more personal questions, but it still bothered me that I had seemingly passed this patient off as a simple, typical older gentleman. In fact, he had a huge back story and was a very active, caring man.

I think that I lost my opportunity that day. However, this realization actually provided me an opportunity. It reminded me that with all patients I would have from that point forward, I should be sure to get to know them as individuals. After all, each of us has special talents and things that make us unique from one another. As nurses, it is these individual characteristics that we must learn about our patients in order to provide the best care possible.

After my first day, I also recorded this in my reflection:

"My first 'real' clinical was very exciting and fun. Admittedly, I was a bit worried about being in a new facility, not knowing staff, and, in general, being in an unknown situation. However, the experience turned out to be very rewarding."

And clinical days from that point on would be "exciting and fun" . . . for the most part, anyway. Where would I go from this point – from this first clinical? I didn't know at the time. But I would realize how special nursing as a profession is as I continued my tenure in nursing school.

Ch. 3:
Notes on Nursing

Back in the classroom, I was quickly learning just how much nurses actually have to know and how much autonomy they have in the medical setting.

Nursing in general has come a long way since Florence Nightingale wrote her *Notes on Nursing* in 1859. It has flourished into a *profession* with a significant knowledge base, its own governing body, and set standards of practice. While many nursing programs were historically diploma or associate's degree programs, the newest trend has been toward bachelor's degree programs for nursing, and several studies have suggested that increasing the education level of nurses contributes to better patient outcomes (see for example Aiken, Clarke, Cheung, Sloane & Silber, 2003, which was published in the *Journal of the American Medical Association*). Further, the Institute of Medicine (2010) has called for nurses to be "full partners, with physicians and other health care professionals, in redesigning health care in the United States" and also stated that nurses should "achieve higher levels of education and training through an improved education system that promotes seamless academic progression" (p. 4).

However, contrary to true nursing practice, the lay public seems to commonly see nursing in the archaic framework that existed in Nightingale's time. I do not blame them for this lack of understanding; most television shows and movies present a certain stereotyped image of nursing, and so unless a person has extensive experience working in health care or being a patient/family member of a patient, it is unlikely that he or she has had the opportunity to truly understand nursing.

Nightingale focused largely on the patient's environment – the level of light, cleanliness, ventilation and other similar topics. It was her belief that by improving these environmental conditions, it would be possible to help the patient heal or stay healthy. She believed that a less-than-adequate environment was a direct cause of disease.

When I have talked with others about nursing, some of them ask me why I would want to be a nurse. They bring up many of the ideas that were prominent in Nightingale's framework for nursing, including keeping patients' rooms clean and changing beds. Many people ask me why I would want to clean people up after they have been incontinent and deal with bodily wastes. While these are indeed some concerns that nursing addresses, and a very important part that should not be forgotten by nurses, nursing is about so much more than many realize.

I grew up with a rather superficial understanding of nursing. To be quite honest, I never gave nurses enough credit. I did not think it was really "hard" to be a nurse, nor did I realize the vast amount of knowledge nurses have. I greatly underestimated the level of critical thinking that is involved in nursing, as well. While I was always interested in medical topics, most of that medical "knowledge" came from television shows such as *ER* and M*A*S*H. Sure, they were entertaining shows, but I was not able to see all of the behind-the-scenes issues that nurses deal with on a daily basis; all I saw was nurses listening to what physicians told them and having intimate relationships with their colleagues. I did not see nurses stopping a physician to advocate for a patient or a nurse holding a patient's hand as the patient cried because he or she had no family left.

Undoubtedly, there are a lot of "behind-the-scenes issues" that the general public does not understand. Perhaps by answering the following question, the true scope of nursing will be put into perspective: Why do patients get admitted to the hospital or a "nursing home"; why can't a patient just go home? The answer to this question is that these patients need *nursing* care. Sure, the patient may also be seen by other medical professionals, and the nurses are frequently operating under physicians' orders, but the reason patients are admitted is that they need an IV started or need close monitoring of their vital signs or they have many wounds that need to be carefully managed, among other reasons. Thinking about the sort of care that is delivered in the hospital setting especially reveals the breadth of knowledge nurses utilize and the scope of practice in which nurses provide care.

While there are a countless number of examples, perhaps the idea of autonomy in nursing is at the forefront of exemplifying how special nursing care is. Nurses make many independent decisions on a daily basis, not requiring a physician present to say "do this" or "do that."

For example, patients that are likely to experience pain after a certain procedure may be prescribed several medications to help with pain. Generally, these medications may come from different classes and act differently in the body; they also frequently address different levels of pain. The medications are prescribed under *pro re nata* (as the situation arises) or "PRN" status. In other words, these medications are only given when patients need them, and the decision to give these medications and which medications to give largely rests on the shoulders of nurses. For example, a physician may prescribe acetaminophen (Tylenol), hydrocodone/acetaminophen (Norco) and morphine IV, all PRN. While these medications are all analgesics – that is, they help reduce pain – they each treat differing levels of pain, and they each have side effects. If the patient has these three medications ordered and reports pain, it is up to the nurse to assess the patient's level of pain and make a nursing judgment about what level of pain medication is needed.

Further, the nurse will also use the understanding that these medications have different lengths of action. That is, each of the three pain medications stays in the patient's body and stays active a different amount of time. Therefore, if the patient's pain is significant, the nurse may choose to give more than one pain medication, spaced at appropriate intervals to provide proper pain management. At the same time, the nurse has to keep in mind that the Tylenol and Norco both contain acetaminophen, and the daily maximum dosage for acetaminophen is 4 grams, though for many patients no more than 3 grams is preferred. (Patients with liver and other metabolic problems may not be permitted to take any amount of acetaminophen, primarily due to the toll acetaminophen takes on the liver's cells.) Thus, nurses have to be cognizant of how much Tylenol and how much Norco the patient has received in a day to make sure that the patient does not receive too much acetaminophen.

In her *Notes on Nursing*, Nightingale did not address another one of the most prominent function of nurses today – therapeutic communication and more specifically the nurse-patient relationship. Early on in my nursing education, during my introductory 202 nursing course, we learned how important communicating with patients is and what good communication entails. Nurses spend a lot of time talking with patients, family members and their co-workers, and being able to talk with all of them in an empathic way that conveys concern is of utmost importance. Nobody wants to talk to a nurse that is cold and seems unconcerned. Further, nurses need to be able to develop a trusting relationship very quickly with patients. It is not easy to find out what drug a patient took if that patient does not trust the nurse. When nurses have mastered proper therapeutic communication techniques, they are frequently able to evoke this sort of information from patients. When I got to my mental health clinical rotation, I really learned how important therapeutic communication is in nursing.

In addition to her rather lengthy writings about the patient's environment, in her initial writings, Nightingale distinguished nursing from the medical profession (primarily physicians). While nursing is indeed different from medicine, that does not mean that nursing and medicine do not work hand-in-hand to take care of patients and provide optimal outcomes. The interdisciplinary work that occurs especially in the hospital setting is invaluable and should never be underestimated in importance. While nurses, physicians, social workers, pharmacists, clerks, phlebotomists, radiology technologists, food service associates, registrars, nursing technicians, and all other personnel may sometimes get "annoyed" with one another, the possibilities are endless when all health care professionals and staff members work together collaboratively to take care of patients.

Ch. 4:
George, the Dog

Not all lessons learned from clinical experiences take a serious tone. It was my second week of clinical, and my patient was just about ready to be discharged. This 80-year-old female had been admitted about a week prior with severe pneumonia, which required her to be on some potent IV antibiotics. She was doing much better, however, and her physician was ready to give her the "okay" to be sent back to her assisted living facility.

Her main problem area when I was taking care of her was the fact that she had significant dementia – specifically Alzheimer's disease.

Alzheimer's disease is a rather insidious disease that affects not only memory but also the ability to carry out daily tasks, such as brushing teeth or shaving. It almost exclusively affects adults over age 65, but researchers are now learning that the onset of the disease may be decades earlier. This disease is coming into focus as another significant threat to older adults. Because older adults are living longer, we are beginning to see more and more patients developing the disease. Further, there is a lot more to learn about this condition, and much of the pathophysiology of Alzheimer's is not fully understood. Thus, treatment options are fairly limited, as compared with other diseases.

When I walked into the patient's room for the first time, I was not sure what to expect. Having looked at her chart the evening before, I knew that she had Alzheimer's disease and that her memory deficits were obvious, but I had never worked with any patients with this disease before. I introduced myself in the usual fashion. "Hi, my name is John, and I am a nursing student . . ."

She smiled up at me, beaming from her bed, looking frail but full of spirit. She reported that she was feeling good and that she "guessed" she slept well the night before. I then asked her the classic questions to assess how alert and oriented she was: What is your name? Where are you? What year is it? I could have asked her what month it was, but I figured if she knew what year it was, we would be doing well. She knew her name, but that was about it. She thought that she was in her house and that it was 1999. She was only around a decade off.

I also noticed a small stuffed dog sitting on the bedside table. I wondered if she could remember who gave her the dog and if it had a name, so I asked her. She responded that she thought her daughter had given it to her but that she was not entirely sure. As for the name, no, the dog did not have a name. However, what came next I was not expecting. "Why don't you name it? It needs a name," she said.

While I knew that nursing involved many different roles, I saw nowhere in the job description that I would be naming stuffed animals. However, in the moment, it was all about the patient.

I responded by asking her if she wanted to give it a name instead, but she insisted that I have the privilege of assigning a name to this eight inch long, stuffed dog. "I guess I'll call it George," I responded.

Why George? I have no idea. It was the name that came to me right at that moment. She was happy with it, though.

In hind sight, I probably should have given it a different name. Her husband had died just two months prior, and I was not sure what his name was. I was concerned that, if her husband's name had been George and she remembered that, she might ask where her husband was. That's not a comfortable conversation to have with a patient that does not remember her husband is actually deceased.

This was not the case, however, so I dodged that bullet.

The rest of the morning was fairly uneventful. I spent the majority of the time helping to orient the patient to her surroundings and assisting her with her meals.

At the end of the day, I guess the overall lesson learned from that day was that a nurse never knows what he or she will be called to do. In this case, the task was fairly simple and light-hearted. In other situations, the calling can be more serious . . .

Ch. 5:
The Nursing Process

It was about one third of the way through the semester when we all shuffled into our stuffy classroom. It was still very cold outside, and there was snow on the ground, but the room felt like an oven, making learning theoretical material about as difficult as climbing Mt. Everest. Little did we know that today we would be learning about one of the most important foundational components of nursing.

Professor Davis made her way into the room and announced that we would be learning about the nursing process that day. The nursing process? Many of us had read about it in our reading assignment for that day, but it still seemed so technical. Would we really be going through a bunch of steps with every single patient we took care of? Why did we need to be so methodical? As we would learn, we did (and do in our everyday practice as RNs) use the nursing process – maybe not consciously or by having to think about it, but we did (and do) use it. It is essentially the framework for nursing practice and helps to foster critical thinking about patient care problems. This process is also essentially the outline for a care plan, which is discussed later. The nursing process follows five major steps, though some professors add a sixth dimension. The nursing process includes:

1. Assessment
2. Diagnosis
3. Outcomes/Planning
4. Implementation
5. Evaluation
6. Documentation (unofficial sixth step)

Looking at these steps, if you are not familiar with nursing, you might say, "Diagnosis? Wait, isn't that something a physician does? What about planning? I thought physicians and other health care providers plan care for patients."

However, nursing has its own set of diagnoses and its own special interventions. The following discussion will briefly discuss the nursing process and give you an idea of what goes into the care of a patient utilizing this process.

Assessment

As the name might indicate, assessment involves obtaining information from the client – both subjective (information that comes from the patient) and objective (information that the nurse observes). Assessment data includes information such as blood pressure, pulse and temperature, along with descriptions from the patient about pain or how hard it is to breathe. As the American Nurses Association (2012) points out, assessment is not always as simple as it seems and includes more than just information that is physiologically based, including "psychological, sociocultural, spiritual, economic, and life-style factors." If a nurse finds out that a patient is not adhering to his medication regimen exactly as prescribed, for example, that nurse may look into the situation in more depth and try to find out why the patient is not taking these medications correctly. Perhaps the patient does not have enough money to pay for the medication, or maybe he does not fully understand the medication regimen. In any case, the assessment portion of the nursing process helps to ferret out this sort of information. (Of interesting note, a lack of proper adherence to medication regimens may come at a cost of almost $300 billion – yes billion with a "b" – per year, according to the New England Healthcare Institute, 2009.) Thus, the nurse's ability to identify nonadherence and then to figure out the root cause of the nonadherence is very important. This is merely one reason why assessment (and the role of nursing in general) is important.

Diagnosis

While people may tend to think of diagnoses in terms of "cancer," "heart failure," or "appendicitis," these are medical diagnoses – distinctly different than nursing diagnoses. Nursing utilizes its own diagnoses, generally based on the North American Nursing Diagnosis Association (NANDA). Every few years, this organization publishes an updated, evidence-based list of nursing diagnoses that is utilized by nurses and organizations across North America.

Nursing diagnoses include those such as "acute pain," "activity intolerance," "risk for bleeding," and "impaired tissue integrity." These nursing diagnoses are able to be specifically addressed by nursing interventions and are generally direct results of (or potential problems associated with) other medical conditions. While a registered professional nurse cannot "treat" appendicitis, since RNs cannot prescribe medications or perform surgery, they can treat the acute pain that comes along with it. They administer pain medications as ordered and, after surgery, may address impaired tissue integrity by carefully taking care of the incision sites.

In addition to the diagnosis phrase, a "complete" diagnosis also includes an "as evidenced by" segment which is essentially a list of assessment data that supports the diagnosis. The "secondary to" statement is the medical diagnosis or reason for the diagnosis. For example, the patient's full diagnosis may be "acute pain related to incisional wound, tissue injury secondary to surgical procedure."

While this is a rather simplified explanation of nursing diagnoses, I think that it gives you an adequate understanding of what nursing diagnoses entail and how they differ from medical diagnoses.

Outcomes/Planning

Once a diagnosis (or, as is the case for almost every patient, more than one diagnosis) is made, outcome goals are established, and the nurse must plan how he or she is going to help address the problem the patient has. These goals that are established are both short-term and long-term, and they must be measurable. For example, an outcome may be that we want the patient to be able to walk, but how far do we want him or her to walk? We must be specific and say our goal is that "The patient will walk 50 feet without becoming short of breath by the end of the clinical day on 10/24/2014," or something along those lines. Notice that this goal also includes a deadline for this to occur – the end of clinical on 10/24.

Implementation
Implementation means, well, the nurse puts the care plan into action and addresses the patient's problem area(s).

Evaluation
Like implementation, evaluation is exactly what the name suggests. During the evaluation, the nurse must determine whether the outcomes have been met and whether any changes need to be made to the care plan.

Documentation (the unofficial sixth step)
While documentation is not considered an official part of the nursing process, just about every nursing student can tell you that documentation is an absolutely critical component of nursing. It is ingrained in our brains, after all. As the saying that almost every nursing student can recite reads, "If it isn't documented, it didn't happen" (or some variation of this sentence). In other words, even if the nurse performs some intervention, even as simple as changing the bed, if it is not documented in the patient's chart (generally on the electronic chart in the computer) it did not happen. If a case were taken to court, even if the nurse did in fact do something he or she was supposed to, if the chart does not reflect that, legally, the nurse has no recourse.

I do not mean to bore you with this more technical information about nursing school. True, it isn't narrative prose that is particularly interesting, but I think that it does help to provide a picture of what nursing really is. It is much more than just learning specific tasks (starting IVs, taking blood pressures, etc.), and it involves a great deal of knowledge and critical thinking.

Ch. 6:
"I don't want to do this anymore."

I went to the hospital the night before and glanced at the assignment sheet to see what patient I would be taking care of the next day.

"Mr. Smith, 82, male" the board read.

I logged onto the computer and pulled up the patient's hospital summary as well as history and physical. I made it a custom of reading the summary and history and physical first, as this gave me a pretty good overview of the patient. The history and physical contains the vital information about the patient, including the patient's general health, medical and surgical history, social history, family history and other information of importance.

After the summary and history and physical, I would look at the more specific, finite details, such as lab values, assessment findings and radiology test results.

The patient I would have the next day looked to be somewhat of a challenge. He was 82 years old and had a significant medical history, including hypertension (high blood pressure), hyperlipidemia (high cholesterol), diabetes mellitus type 2, chronic obstructive pulmonary disease (COPD), congestive heart failure, hyperthyroidism, kidney failure, a fairly significant heart rhythm abnormality, multiple episodes of cancer with chemotherapy and, to top it all off, severe visual impairment. He had a very lengthy surgical history as well. Originally, he had been admitted with severe difficulty breathing and an exacerbation of his heart failure. The patient's ejection fraction, a measure of how well the heart muscle is working, was only 15%. Essentially, this meant that, when the patient's left ventricle (chamber on the left side of the heart that is responsible for sending blood out into the body) contracted, only 15% of the blood in the ventricle was actually pumped out into the body. The patient was extremely weak, and his COPD was acting up as well. They were having a terrible time keeping his oxygen levels up, and the smallest amount of movement caused this patient's oxygen level to plummet.

In short, this patient was a very, very sick man. Further, at this point, he was still considered a "full code." Knowing a patient's code status is always important, as patients should have their wishes met, whether that means they want nothing done or everything done. If this patient took a turn for the worse, which was certainly *not* out of the question, and stopped breathing, or his heart stopped beating, he would be fully resuscitated. CPR would be performed, and he would potentially be ventilated by a machine with oxygen.

As I was looking at the electronic medical record, a nurse or nursing technician (I can't remember which now), walked by and asked me who I was going to have. After informing her that I had Mr. Smith in room such and such, her response was, "Oh. Good luck. He's a tough one." Great. I was sure the next day of clinical was going to go just marvelously. Two things were going through my mind: 1) Thanks, Prof. Brown. Could you have given me a harder patient? 2) Great. This should be interesting (in the most sarcastic tone possible).

See, at this point in my nursing school career, I was still hoping for the easiest patients. Because I was so new to everything, I was more scared to do things and didn't want to be challenged. Of course, as the weeks and semesters went on and I began to be more comfortable in my skin as a nursing student, I became more confident and began to seek out the difficult patients and the nursing tasks that I had not done yet (a milk and molasses enema might be the most outrageous task I every sought out).

I knew that this clinical day was going to be a bit more challenging than my previous, when I spent the day doing fairly basic tasks and naming a stuffed animal, but I did not quite expect it to be as unique as it indeed ended up.

The next morning, I met this patient. He was every bit as sick as his medical record made him sound, and his family was present in the room with him. There he was, lying in his bed with very pale skin and sad, depressed-looking eyes. He had the head of his bed elevated at about 40 degrees and had multiple pillows propping up his arms and upper body. He had a Foley catheter running into his bladder and also had two separate IV lines running into his arms.

While I was taking the patient's blood pressure, the family began talking with the patient about his wishes. I could feel the tension in the room. The chaplain had been by the evening before talking with the patient about filling out an advanced directive that would allow him to state whether he would want to be resuscitated if it came to that. It became obvious very quickly, however, that what the patient wanted and what the family wanted were two different things.

The daughter was telling the patient, "We don't want to sit here and just watch you give up," but the patient was tired of fighting.

"I'm just tired, and I don't want to do this anymore," he said.

With just this short dialogue between the family members, I was already feeling the emotions coming out inside of me. Not only was I concerned that the family was seemingly minimizing the patient's wishes, but I was thinking about my own grandparents and how I might feel if they were in this same situation.

I finished up vital signs as the family continued their conversation. One of the other children was giving his father a bit more say. "If that's what you really want Dad, I think we should go with it," he stated.

I left the room to return the vital sign machine to its proper place and saw this patient's nurse in the hallway. I stopped and asked her if she knew anything about the advanced directive the patient was to fill out, and she told me that apparently the doctor was supposed to be talking with the patient and family about writing a "do not resuscitate order" for the patient later that morning. This order would prohibit life saving measures from being taken if the patient stopped breathing, or his heart stopped beating. I was happy to hear that the physician was to be involved, as I thought that what was really going on with the family was likely denial. This patient was in bad shape, and the multiple illnesses this patient had gave him a very grim outlook. However, some of the family members wanted the patient to continue to fight, even though he was ready to be done fighting. He was simply exhausted.

It was already impossible for him to get out of bed to do anything. He did not even have enough energy to feed himself. Perhaps if the physician spoke with the family, they would be more realistic about this patient's chances for a meaningful life.

When I re-entered the room to perform my full head-to-toe assessment, the family asked me a surprising question: "What do you think about Dad's condition," they asked.

This question, without a doubt, took me back. I was shocked that they were asking for *my* opinion, since I was "only" a nursing student. What did I really know about this patient's chances? Yes, I "knew my stuff" and was able to provide safe patient care, but who was I to give them information about their Dad's condition? Further, I had only been in the room one time before, so they were clearly putting trust in me simply because of my position as a nursing student, not because of anything I said the time before when I was in the room.

Looking back, of course, I realize that this is what nursing is about. The nurse is there as a patient advocate, definitely, but nurses also help take care of the family, as well. I was not very confident in my own abilities at that time. After all, I had only been in this clinical course for a few weeks at this point, and I did not have much direct patient care experience.

This question also made me realize that I was in a position of great power. Here I was, a mere sophomore in college, being asked about a patient's chances at a meaningful life. What other college students were asked this sort of question? I thought for a very long time after this event about the amount of trust patients and their families put in me. To this day, it humbles me to realize how much patients and their families trust my colleagues and me. We are indeed privileged to be able to provide the care that we do to patients.

When I had composed myself, I admittedly took the easy way out. My answer was a simple, "I really don't think I am in a position to say much about it. I haven't been taking care of your dad that long, so that's probably a better question for his physician." They accepted this answer, and I was glad. If I had to do it all over, I would have also then made sure that the families concern was communicated with the physician.

Later that morning, the physician did come by, and the patient did get his do not resuscitate order. The family also left a little later in the morning to take a rest, and I was able to have some one-on-one time with the patient. Though it sounds rather poetic, this patient looked and sounded so relieved. By just being able to have his wishes honored, he stated that he felt at ease.

"You know," he said, "they just don't want to let go of me, but I've had my time here on this earth. I know that I'm going upstairs to see the big man, and I'm going to be just fine." Apparently, the patient had explained this same logic to his children earlier when the physician was in, and this is what really helped them see the patient's point of view.

Knowing that he would not have to suffer any longer when the time came gave the patient a sense of choice and control that he hadn't had. For so many patients, this is of utmost importance. Feeling out of control is perhaps one of the most common concerns of patients, and I have heard it over and over. When patients feel that they have no say in what happens to them, their anxiety levels rise astronomically. He didn't want a tube inserted into his airway, and he did not want nearly every rib in his body to be broken when CPR was performed on him. No, he wanted to be able to die peacefully. He was realistic about his irreversible medical conditions and had lived a good life. He wanted to be able to have a peaceful death on his own terms. Because of his belief in a life with his savior, he was at peace with death.

To this day, I do not know what happened to this patient. I know that he lived the rest of that day. Whether he lived one more day or another year, he was comfortable with the life he had lived and the decision he made.

Ch. 7:
Wrapping Up Semester One

"The days and weeks seem like they drag on, but the semester seems so short." I got used to this statement, and I said it a time or two during my time in nursing school. It was hard to believe how fast the first semester went.

When we started the semester, it seemed as though our time in Intro Practicum in Nursing and Health Assessment would never end. However, in this first sixteen weeks, we had all learned a great deal – not only theoretical knowledge but also a lot about each other and the profession of nursing in general.

We started with 32 students, but by the end of the semester, only 28 advanced due to the rigor of the course. (We had actually started with over 50 at the very beginning of school, during freshman year, but we lost several students to other majors, and some dropped out of college all together.)

Each of us got to know one other better during the semester, but we still had not grown as close as we would eventually become. The next semester would be even more demanding. Not only would we be in classes like Intro to Sociology, Biology of Birds, Ireland in America and History Since 1865, but we would be moving on to NU 410, Mental Health-Mental Illness Nursing, as well as NU 315, Pathophysiologic Concepts for Nursing. Little did I know, but this semester would be one of tremendous growth for me as a nursing student and individual, and I would find that pathophysiology was my forte.

PART II:
Mental Health-Mental Illness Nursing

Ch. 8:
A New Focus

Intro Practicum in Nursing had ended in May, so I was able to enjoy a nice three months before returning to school. A lot happened between the semesters. Perhaps most importantly, I began working as a phlebotomist at my local hospital. I spent the summer searching for veins and drawing blood from patients across the lifespan, in both the outpatient and inpatient setting. I really enjoyed the high-paced nature of the emergency department but also appreciated working with older adults on the transitional care unit.

I would continue to work in the lab throughout my time in nursing school "per diem" (as needed). I tended to work some weekends and during my holiday breaks. Not only did this "job" give me a little extra money, but it provided me with experience working in the hospital setting and working with the interdisciplinary team. I put job in quotations because it was not really a job. I really enjoyed going to work because I had such a great team to work with. My two and a half years at Taylorville Memorial Hospital were truly wonderful, and I will never forget the lessons I learned and the people I met.

This semester, the focus would be on "mental illness." I had never been a fan of the word mental illness since our psychopathology class when we discussed the various "mental illnesses." I tended (and still do) to prefer the term "psychobiologic illness" – a biologic illness that simply resides in the brain tissue.

Much like the previous semester, our first few weeks were spent in intense lectures. On Tuesday and Thursday, we spent what would be clinical time in lecture, but they did cut the time back somewhat. We only had four and a half hour long lectures. At least during this time they gave us a couple bathroom breaks.

On the first substantive day of lecture, we learned all about the nurse-patient relationship and the phases of this relationship, as originally outlined by Hildegard Peplau, the "mother of psychiatric nursing." One of the overall key concepts for the semester was learning how to talk to patients and how to do so in a therapeutic, helpful way. Talking with some of the most vulnerable patients and assisting them to work towards being healthier would be very important.

"During this semester you will learn how to ask people if they are feeling suicidal and how to do so in a way that is non-threatening," one professor remarked. "You might feel uncomfortable asking this question, but it's an absolutely necessary component of nursing, especially with patients suffering from a mental illness," she said.

As I mentioned, mental illness is really a psychobiologic illness. A lot of stigma still surrounds these sorts of illnesses, and people tend to think that these psychobiologic illnesses fit into their own category. However, consider the following:

Rob is having trouble getting out of bed in the morning. Life is just not as happy as it used to be, and he is stressed out about everything going on in his life. He feels depressed and just has no energy to enjoy life. No matter what he does – focusing on the positive, trying to get exercise when he can – he just cannot force himself to feel happy. He decides to go to his physician and is prescribed an antidepressant, along with counseling. When he gets back home to his apartment that he shares with three other college roommates, he makes no mention of the medication and simply keeps his new diagnosis of depression secret. His mood improves over time, and through the use of counseling and medication, he is able to recover from his depression. However, because of the stigma of mental illness, he has not shared this diagnosis or his medication information with anyone.

Lindsey has terrible sinus pressure and has recently discovered she has a fever. She complains to her roommates about this condition and ends up making a trip to health services, where she is prescribed an antibiotic. When she returns home to her housemates, she happily informs them that she has some medication to "take care of this sinus infection." She is pleased to know that she will soon be feeling better, and she doesn't mind sharing this information with her friends/family.

The two previous scenarios illustrate how mental illnesses are stigmatized in society and also how "mental illnesses" are separated into a separate category from "physical illnesses." However, science is largely proving that mental problems/disorders have, at their root, a biological cause – both genetic and immediate (neurotransmitters, most of the time, which are chemicals that control brain function which translates to our overall emotions/behaviors). Both types of illnesses – depression and a sinus infection – are due to something going wrong somewhere in the body. Looking at the previous scenarios, in one case, neurotransmitters are becoming imbalanced (depression), and Rob cannot control the way he feels. In the other case (sinus infection), Lindsey's defense mechanisms have failed, and she has fallen victim to bacteria and come down with an infection. Either way, the diseases are out of their control. They didn't choose their diseases.

Why should people be afraid to say that they are taking an anti-depressant, an anti-anxiety agent, or an anti-psychotic? Why? At the moment it is because people are afraid others will judge them – that others will think that they are "weak" or something along those lines. It's not true, though. Do we look at someone with cancer and tell them to buck up and get better? I don't think so. Likewise, we shouldn't tell a person with generalized anxiety disorder, major depression, schizophrenia, or post-traumatic stress disorder to buck up and get better.

Furthermore, are psychiatrists and neurologists really looking at the same things a lot of times? Certainly they have different focuses right now, but if we know there is such a strong biological link with mental illness and that mental illness is a disease process, just like all other diseases, why do we have separate names for these people? Really, shouldn't they all be neurologists? Instead, we give the "crazy people" to the psychiatrists (or the "shrinks" if you like), and the neurologists get the "normal" people with problems with their brains, such as those with epilepsy or brain trauma. Of course, I would argue that there isn't a whole lot of difference between someone with epilepsy and someone with schizophrenia.

Being around patients diagnosed with mental illnesses is a lot different than many might imagine. It's not really that scary, and after I adjusted to the setting, I was never really afraid that someone was going to attack me unexpectedly. There are tense moments at times, but it's actually a much calmer and more peaceful environment than many medical-surgical units. Is it hard to believe? Probably – probably because society has projected certain views about those with mental illness and psychiatric hospitals/behavioral health units.

As you read the next several chapters, try to put yourself not only in my place as a nursing student but also in the place of the patients I discuss and the situations I experienced.

Ch. 9:
Welcome to the Behavioral Health Unit

I was very apprehensive about starting clinical this semester. I had only seen the stereotypical images of psychiatric (also called behavioral health) units in the media – such as in the infamous 1975 film *One Flew Over the Cuckoo's Nest*, featuring Jack Nicholson. I was expecting to enter a world where I would be constantly threatened. I was definitely wrong, though.

For this clinical experience, some of us had to drive about 40 minutes to a hospital in another city. While some clinical groups in our class were assigned to locations in Decatur, I was lucky enough to be able to commute this distance each week. When I say lucky, I am not actually being sarcastic. Driving allowed a few advantages.

First, because we had to devote almost an hour and a half and a good half tank of gas to driving, clinical for this semester was only one day per week and lasted around nine hours. This allowed for a more realistic experience on the unit, since we had a lot more time to spend with the patients.

Second, I was able to "shoot the breeze" with a couple of my fellow nursing students on the way to clinical and on the trip back to Decatur, as I carpooled with two of the other students in my class, Ian and Richie. We had some great conversations and got to know a lot more about each others' lives.

And, finally, being able to drive gave me time that I could not really be doing anything else but sitting and thinking or talking. In a very busy semester, this commute time gave me some forced "relaxation" – relaxation that I may not otherwise have afforded myself and time that was most definitely needed.

Clinical started at noon this semester, so there was no waking up at the crack of dawn this semester. On our first day, I woke up at a little after 10:00 AM and began to go through the usual routine of hygiene and putting on my clothes. Instead of wearing our uniforms, this semester, we would be wearing business casual attire.

Ian whipped into the parking spot just before 11:00 AM, and I made my way out to his car, acknowledging Richie as I slid into the back seat. I think I said something along the lines of, "This should be fun," in a very sarcastic manner. I was seriously terrified of what my day would be like. I just knew something I said would "set off" one of the patients.

Neither Richie nor Ian were too keen on this first clinical day either. We would be working on an inpatient behavioral health unit. To even be admitted to the hospital patients must be at risk for harming themselves or others or lack the ability to care for themselves, so we knew these patients were very sick.

As we made our way west on the interstate, we continued to discuss what our day would be like. We shared our ideas of what the unit would look like and what kind of patients we would be working with. "I'm sure it looks a lot like a prison," Richie said, and Ian and I both seemed to agree with this statement, as it seemed logical to us. In a lot of movies and television shows, it seemed that patients with mental illnesses were simply locked up and forgotten about. We would find out that this was not the case anymore, though in the not-so-distant past, patients with mental illnesses were treated more similar to criminals than persons with a biological problem.

We parked in a parking lot about a block from the hospital, which would become the routine. Sometimes we had to make several passes through to find a spot.

Once we hopped out of Ian's white sports car and drug our heavy nursing bags out of the back seat, we made our way up to the hospital. On this first day, it almost felt like slow motion walking up to the building. We were supposed to meet the rest of our class in the lobby area of the hospital, and when we walked in, there were already a few of our classmates there. They looked like us – white as ghosts, appearing as though they could, in the words of my fourth grade teacher, "upchuck," at any moment.

Our professor, Dr. Keller, was also there. She stood at least six feet tall (it seemed to us to be about seven feet) with deep red hair and an average build. If not for her calm and soothing voice, she would have been an intimidating individual. But it was that comfort that Dr. Keller was able to project that made being in her clinical group more pleasant and also what made her an excellent psychiatric-mental health nurse.

She seemed slightly amused that we were all so nervous – probably because she knew what we would actually be facing on the behavioral health unit, and what we would be facing was far, far from the visions we had conjured up.

Once everyone in our group had arrived, we made our way up to the pre-conference room, which was actually the waiting room for electroconvulsive therapy (ECT) treatments, also called "shock therapy" by some. When many people think of ECT, they may flash back to images from a movie such as *One Flew Over the Cuckoo's Nest*. Now, however, this treatment method has become much more humane and does not even remotely resemble the scene portrayed in the movie. We had clinical on Thursday, and no treatments were performed on this day of the week.

As we sat there in the waiting room, nervous as all get out, I couldn't help but think of the patients that came to receive their first ECT treatments – uncertain of what they were about to face, just as we were quite unsure of what we would be facing.

"So, how is everyone feeling," Dr. Keller asked us.

Sitting in a circle, we just kind of looked around at each other like we wanted to hurl. "I'm terrified I'm going to do something wrong," one of my fellow students said.

My concern for a long time was that I was going to "set off" a patient – say the wrong word and send the patient into a downward spiral of explosive anger. We had learned in lecture, after all, how important therapeutic communication is when creating, maintaining and ending the nurse-patient relationship.

A week prior to this first clinical day, Dr. Keller had given us a sheet to fill out, with several questions measuring our level of anxiety for this clinical rotation. We were asked to rate our anxiety level on a scale from 0 to 10, 10 being the highest level of anxiety we had ever felt; I rated my anxiety at an 8 at the beginning of the semester.

After telling Dr. Keller of my concern, she said, "Do you normally set your friends off when you talk to them?"

At the time, I didn't really understand what she is getting at, but after a few weeks on the unit, I realized what she meant. She was making the point that talking with patients that have a major mental illness is a lot like talking to any other person – there is no reason to be especially afraid of the interaction. If I could just act naturally and use my therapeutic communication skills, I would be just fine.

After some of our initial questions were answered and anxiety levels and imaginations were slightly subdued by the reassurance of Dr. Keller, we began to discuss patients for the clinical day. There were eight of us, and four would be on one part of the unit – the "intensive" side – and four of us would be on another part of the unit – the "step-down" side. Each group would spend half of the semester on the same part of the unit and then switch, so all of us would get to experience both sides of the unit.

The intensive side included patients with more aggressive or acute episodes that tended to be on 15 minute suicide precautions, and some were aggressive, agitated or having active hallucinations and/or delusions. On the step-down side, the patients tended to have a diagnosis of depression without significant hallucinations/delusions, and many of these patients had initially been on the intensive side. Some were also on the unit to receive electroconvulsive therapy. I was assigned to the step-down side for the first part of the semester and the intensive side for the second part of the semester, which I did not mind.

Dr. Keller took a slightly different approach than the previous semester. Instead of assigning us a patient that we had to take, she would pick several patients that would be "good" for students, and it was up to us to decide who was going to take which patient; this allowed us to decide what experiences we still needed. For instance, if we had worked with a few patients with schizophrenia, we would know we needed to select a patient with a different diagnosis the next time. She would give us a quick summary of each patient – their name, age, sex, diagnosis, and a brief summary of what brought the patient in and how they were doing. Then, it was up to us to barter back and forth with the patients. It is a good thing that our clinical group got along well, as we were fair, I think, with each other and the patients we each chose. Once we chose a patient, we would have about an hour to collect information about the patient, including their history and medications.

Especially for the first clinical, I was glad we were able to choose our patient, as it enabled me to pick a patient that I was fairly comfortable with – or as comfortable as I could have been at the time.

Given my affinity for the older adult population, I was looking for the oldest patient possible. I chose Mrs. Trebble, an 83-year-old female with an admitting diagnosis of major depression with suicidal ideation, meaning that she had been thinking about committing suicide.

Once we had all made our selection, Dr. Keller said that it was time to head to the unit. We all picked up our nursing bags and headed slowly – very slowly – towards the door. I think all of our stomachs were churning faster than a washing machine on steroids at that moment. It was not a very long walk to the unit, and we had to be buzzed in.

As we made our way down the hallway, it became very apparent that this unit was not designed like a prison. No, it was actually very brightly lit, and the patient rooms looked nearly identical to typical hospital rooms. There were even several areas where patients could congregate and talk with each other as well as areas for various activities. Seeing the layout of the unit caused an initial shifting of my understanding of what behavioral health units are really like.

We put our belongings away in the staff break room and headed to report to listen to information on our patient. After finding out that the patient seemed to be doing okay and that she had not been having any feelings of suicide, I made my way to the nurses' station to begin looking up patient information. While looking at her history, I found out that in addition to her depression, she was suffering from Alzheimer's disease.

Mrs. Trebble's medical history, other than the Alzheimer's and depression, was fairly unremarkable, other than a tonsillectomy and adenoidectomy she had as a child. She did have several medications for her depression and dementia, however. Because her medications did not seem to be working to control her feelings of suicide, she was receiving ECT as well.

After looking up the various medications the patient was on and obtaining background information on her, I picked up my clipboard, took a deep breath and made my way down the hallway to Mrs. Trebble's room. It felt like I had bricks in my shoes with every step I took, but I eventually made it the several room-lengths down the hallway.

I knocked on her door, as we had been taught to do and then walked in. Mrs. Trebble looked up from her bed. She had been reading a book. She gave me a half smile, though I seemed to sense some pain in her expression – not physical pain but rather mental pain. "Hello," I said. "My name is John, and I am a nursing student. I'm here to work with you today, along with your nurse."

"Oh, hi," she said.

Initially, she did not have a lot to say, and she was pretty much just responding to the questions I asked her, not uncommon for patients with a diagnosis of depression and many other psychobiologic illnesses. I made some small talk and took her vital signs, trying to begin the therapeutic nurse-patient relationship. Once I had completed the vital signs and asked her how she was feeling, I asked her if there was anything she wanted to talk about or work on during my time with her, and she responded by saying, "No. It's just nice to talk."

I informed her that I would be back in just a little bit to talk with her. I also began to formulate my plan for the day. I wanted to spend time talking with her since I had the time and since that seemed to be what she wanted. I also wanted to get her out of her room and encourage her to meander out to the public area and possibly interact with other patients on the unit. At the very least, we could work on a puzzle.

After charting her vital signs in the computer and discussing my initial plan of care for the day with Dr. Keller, I walked back to Mrs. Trebble's room. I was feeling a bit more comfortable at this point, since I had seen that my patient was not psychotic and seemed to be a very pleasant woman.

Further, the unit itself had been much calmer than I had anticipated, and I was happy about that.

We spent the next couple hours discussing a variety of topics, and Mrs. Trebble really enjoyed having someone to talk to. And it was not just a "shoot-the-breeze" type conversation, either. The conversation was full of therapeutic communication – allowing the patient to express her feelings, concerns and perceptions. This then allowed me to help provide her with ideas to cope with her Alzheimer's and depression. Sometimes I think that the general public may listen to a conversation between a nurse and patient and just think of it as random chit-chat. However, many times, there is purpose in what the nurse is saying and asking; the more the nurse can understand about the patient's situation, feelings and perceptions, the more effectively the nurse can help the patient.

Pretty early in the conversation, it became apparent that Mrs. Trebble's biggest concern was with her losses created by her Alzheimer's. In her opinion, there was a set event that triggered a worsening of her depression, and she could identify it and explain it as if it happened yesterday.

"I was in town driving. I was to have my hair cut at noon, and I had gotten in my car and pulled out of my driveway," she said. "When I reached the stop sign, I just did not know what to do – whether I should stop or turn or continue on straight. Another car honked at me, and at the time I did not understand why; I just became more upset and confused. Then I totally forgot where I was going and what I was doing and had to pull off to the side of the road and call my daughter."

And perhaps what was most troubling to Mrs. Trebble, aside from the losses she was facing in her daily functioning, was the fact that it was unpredictable. Specifically, she said that she sometimes had a better memory than others and that she could remember some things one day but would totally forget that same information a different day. She still knew her family but was not always able to brush her teeth. She could recall stories, such as the day she got lost in her car, but she could not always remember what she had for breakfast.

"I will pick up my hair brush some days, but then I cannot remember what to do with it," she said in a sad, melancholy tone.

This patient had a special impact on me, as she reminded me a lot of my own grandmother. They were both around the same age, and they enjoyed having their hair cut weekly, going shopping at all of the local stores and researching family history. In cases such as this, it is important for the health professional to prevent countertransference, which essentially means that the nurse becomes emotionally attached to the patient at a level deeper than the normal nurse-patient relationship. It is not always easy to prevent countertransference. After all, it is generally in the nature of a nurse to be very caring and compassionate, but it is best to avoid becoming too emotionally involved.

To see this woman who had a life full of sewing, bingo, visiting friends and community service reduced to uncertainty in her daily life was moving for me. This was not exactly what I was expecting for my first day on the behavioral health unit, but, after all, this was one dimension of mental health and nursing in general.

These patients are not just on the behavioral health unit, either; they are admitted to medical-surgical units after having a ruptured appendix, an intensive care unit after an overdose or to an emergency department with reports of chest pain. You see, in nursing, being able to communicate with a variety of people is essential. No matter where a nurse works, he or she will encounter a multitude of patients, each with their own concerns and unique personalities.

I learned a lot more about Mrs. Trebble during those afternoon hours. She told me about her boyfriend, whom she had been with for many years after her husband died. Her boyfriend had been involved in a motor vehicle accident about one year prior and suffered some significant injuries requiring rehabilitation. This accident and her boyfriend's injuries were yet another assault on her psyche. She told me during our conversation that at one point she was sure she was "not only losing my mind but also my love."

This was all very powerful stuff, and it overwhelmed me to a degree.

"Wow," I thought. "My life isn't that bad." Yes, at the time I was under a lot of stress – from nursing school and the normal stressors of life – but I was not under near the stress many of these patients were under.

I would have this "wow" thinking every week while on the behavioral health unit and with pretty much every patient I worked with from that point on. Working in a hospital in general exposes a person to so much sadness and despair, but it also reveals a lot of hope and joy. I experienced both ends of the spectrum during my time in nursing school.

I had left Mrs. Trebble's room and charted her head to toe assessment in the computer and also had given Dr. Keller an update. When I walked back into her room a little later, Mrs. Trebble was reading a book, or at least that is what it looked like. Specifically, she was reading a Bible.

Though it seemed pretty obvious, I asked her, "What are you reading?"

"Well," she said, "I'm not really reading. I can't ever remember what I've just read, so I don't know why I even try anymore."

Mrs. Trebble had gone from reading a couple novels per week to not being able to remember what happened in the previous chapter.

I found out that she was a very religious woman and had always gone to church every Sunday. At the current time, she was also having trouble coming to terms with her Alzhiemer's and why it was happening to her.

"How could this happen to me?" she asked.

Without a doubt, she was having some spiritual distress. She felt that she had lived a good life and done her best but that she was being punished for some reason.

We discussed her concerns a little longer, and we were able to come up with a couple points of action. I would make sure that the pastoral care team came to see her to discuss her spiritual concerns that were directly related to her religion, and I would also try to locate some religious books that included very short stories with meaningful points. That way, she could continue to read but would not be bogged down in excessive amounts of text that she would soon forget. Luckily, I was able to find one of these books in the collection of books on the unit, so she was able to read that.

After supper with the others in my clinical group, we headed back to the unit. There was not a whole lot of time left in our clinical day – only about another hour and a half. I had some charting to do yet again – a summary of the patient's activities for the day, along with some other general information. Mrs. Trebble was napping upon our return, so I opted to chart for a while.

Terminating the nurse-patient relationship is very important in nursing, so telling patients goodbye and that we wish the best for them is highly valued. I waited a while for her to wake up, and she did about an hour later. When I went in to tell her goodbye, she asked me, in a more or less rhetorical way, not expecting an answer, "What will happen to me? What will I become?"

How in the world was I supposed to answer that question? Of course, I knew the answer deep down. Yes, Alzheimer's is progressive and would eventually cause her to be unable to care for herself. She would likely end up in a skilled care facility and die not knowing who any of her family members were. This is not a pleasant picture. It is, however, the reality of late-stage Alzheimer's.

However, she had time left – time to enjoy her family and friends, and so that is how I answered. "I know it must be very difficult for you, but you definitely have a lot of people that care about you. It's easy for me to see looking at the cards here in your room," I said. I'm not sure if that was the best response, but it was my first day on the behavioral health unit, and I was new to it all.

Almost on cue, Mrs. Trebble's boyfriend, aided by her daughter, walked into her room. I don't know if I would call it a "miracle," per se, but it was darn good timing. I was leaving, but Mrs. Trebble would have her beloved boyfriend and daughter to be with after I left.

I also was able to see Mrs. Trebble's face light up. The last image I have of her, as I was walking out her door, is her giving her boyfriend a peck on the lips and a subsequent smile. This was an uplifting moment for me. Even in her losses, she still had love in her life, and that made me feel good.

Ch. 10:
Electroconvulsive Therapy . . .
and Heart Attacks

I learned a lot on the general side of the behavioral health unit, such as how to talk to people and encourage them to express their feelings. Take Michael Rodriguez, for example. Because there weren't any older adult patients one clinical day, I had chosen him, a 46-year-old male patient with major depressive disorder. He had been receiving ECT, as no other treatments had been successful at reducing his suicidal ideation.

When I heard that this patient was middle-aged, the first though that popped into my head was my own father. He was around the age of my patient, and I wondered what it would be like to work with a patient such as this. Would he have similar interests as my father? Would it cause me to think of my father and what it would be like if my father was suffering the way the patient was? Much like the countertransference that had a risk of occurring with Mrs. Trebble, this risk was also present with Mr. Rodriguez.

After our initial pre-conference discussion, I made my way to the behavioral health unit to listen to report on my patient. I learned that he had been doing well, denying feeling like he wanted to kill himself, and he was to be discharged in the next day or two – depending on his psychiatrist's level of comfort. It looked like my day was going to be fairly straightforward, with no major challenges, other than talking with my patient.

I stood up from my chair after having gathered information from the computer and walked over to the side room to look up medications to be sure I understood all possible side effects and normal dosages, to ensure the patient was on a reasonable dose of all of his medications. Surprisingly, this patient was on relatively few medications, and it did not take me long to look up the various antidepressants and anti-anxiety medications this patient was on.

"Well, I suppose it's time to go see my patient," I thought.

After neatly organizing all of my papers on my clipboard, I made my way down the hallway to Mr. Rodriguez's room. I walked into his room and peered around the corner. He was nowhere to be found. I had a minor panic attack, worrying that my patient had somehow escaped from the unit, not that he was really a major flight risk or anything.

I double checked that he wasn't hiding in the storage closet in his room and then walked down to one of the activity rooms to see if he was there. First, though, I had to stop at the nurses' station to ask what Mr. Rodriguez looked like, since I had never met him before. I really did not want to have to go around to all of the patients potentially in the activity area asking them their names, figuring I would simply worsen paranoia for any of the patients that already thought staff members were working for the Federal Bureau of Investigation and out to get them.

As it turned out, Mr. Rodriguez was by himself, watching television in the back activity room. He was sitting in the reclining chair with his arms relaxed at his side on the armrest. He looked to be his age, with just a slight graying of his hair from it's natural brown. As I walked in, he turned his attention away from the television and glanced up at me with a half smile, though it seemed mostly superficial, as if he knew that it was polite to smile when someone walked in the room but did not really want to smile.

"Hi," I said. "My name is John, and I'm a student nurse from Millikin. One of the nurses told me you are Mr. Rodriguez. Is that correct?"

"Yes, that's me.," he said simply.

After discussing how he was feeling that afternoon and some small talk, it came time for the question that is never extremely easy to ask yet highly necessary. When working with patients on the behavioral health unit (and truthfully patients throughout the hospital), it is absolutely necessary to find out whether they are feeling suicidal or not. In the behavioral health unit, this question was part of the normal assessment, so patients were used to being asked this question, but it was still somewhat awkward.

Here I was, merely a college student, and I was talking to a grown man about whether he felt like harming himself. Later that night, I would be hanging out with friends watching television and surfing Facebook, but here I was, in this moment, having a very serious conversation with a patient.

"It's very important that you stay safe," I said in a very matter of fact way. "Have you felt like harming yourself at all today?"

"No. I've been feeling much better," he said. It was amazing to see the turnaround these patients could do after receiving a course of ECT treatment.

Several students had been able to see a patient admitted one week with a suicide attempt and feeling terrible about themselves only to see that same patient the next week smiling and denying feeling like wanting to hurt themselves after several treatments with ECT. This treatment was used when other treatments were not working or when a patient needed to be treated quickly. It takes several weeks sometimes for antidepressant mediations to take full effect, and when a patient is acutely suicidal, a few weeks is not an option. Thus, when treatment that will have a quick effect is needed, ECT is used.

When talking with Mr. Rodriguez, I quickly realized that it was important to mirror the patient's mood. When I would act too bubbly or happy, he would begin to shut off and not talk much, but each time I brought myself back down and talked in a balanced way, at a slow but steady pace, he was much more willing to express his feelings. He also was very comfortable with silence.

Coming into this semester, our professors had warned us that we would need to become comfortable with silence, as many patients need some time to reflect and process thoughts before talking. Not only do some psychiatric mediations cause processing time to slow a bit, but many patients with neurobiologic problems in general tend to take a while to answer questions. It took me a while, but this idea of taking a moment for patients to process was applicable, and I used it with Mr. Rodriguez a lot.

I would ask a question and pause, allowing him a chance to think and process his answer. With previous patients, I had fallen in the trap of filling this silence with more words. I had wrongly assumed that the patient did not feel comfortable answering my question when, in fact, he or she had just needed a bit more time to process what I had asked.

My days on the general side of the behavioral health unit continued. Today, Dr. Keller had asked us to challenge ourselves a bit more. This was our fifth week on the unit, after all, and she expected us to step out of our comfort zones a little bit more. I had opted for a younger patient this time, a 26-year-old patient with borderline personality disorder (BPD) and anxiety.

Indeed, this would be challenging, I thought. Not only was this patient near my age, but he had a diagnosis of BPD, which is a particularly challenging diagnosis. In fact, when I met with my patient's nurse, she simply said, "Good luck. He's a challenge." That really encouraged me – or actually did the opposite. I wasn't expecting too much for the day. However, I quickly got myself back on track, thinking about my role, which was to help patients to the best of my ability and to come in with no pre-conceived notions.

BPD is characterized by patients that have extreme difficulty in regulating emotion and maintaining relationships. It is common that these patients have a history of traumatic events, such as abuse (many times sexual) during childhood and/or abandonment. (This patient had been abused as a child and also had been left by his mother at age 15.) Frequently, these patients will have angry outbursts and may feel that no one loves them. They often are fairly impulsive and commonly self-injure themselves. Interestingly, even though they have problems maintaining relationships, these patients often prefer to be with a group of people, rather than by themselves.

The beginning of the day went along much like others, quite honestly, with not too much excitement. We had discussed this patient's concerns and feelings and had talked about needs for discharge. The patient had told me how much he disliked his previous nurse but that he absolutely loved me, which I took with a grain of salt. You see, patients with borderline personality disorder frequently use a defense mechanism called "splitting." In short, patients will pit two individuals against each other, favoring one greatly and acting as if the other were the scum of the earth. In this case, I suspected splitting and just accepted the patient's compliment politely. This is one reason that working with patients with BPD is particularly challenging; one minute, a nurse can be the patient's best friend, and the next, the patient can be yelling obscenities and claiming the nurse is terrible. It is vital, though, for staff to realize that splitting is part of the diagnosis and not really part of the person.

Just after returning from our supper break, I had logged on to the computer charting system to double check that I had not missed any charting prior to supper when one of my fellow students, Lia, came hurriedly up to me saying that my patient was in his room asking for help because he couldn't breathe, he was dizzy, his heart was racing, (according to the patient at 200 beats per minute or more), and it felt like his heart was going to beat out of his chest. I quickly jumped up and headed toward the patient's room, telling my professor that my patient was having some problems as I passed her at the nurses' station. She trailed behind but gave me my space, which I was appreciative of.

When I got in the room, Mr. Rodriguez was lying cockeyed on his bed. His left leg was hanging partially off of the bed, and he was looking up at the ceiling, staring. I walked up next to his bed and asked him what was going on, as Lia and I were working together to obtain a set of vital signs from him. He told me what Lia had and added that he just knew that he was dying. However, everything was looking good from a physiologic side. The patient's blood pressure was normal; his pulse was a nice and regular 70 beats per minute; his oxygen saturation was 100% (cannot get any better than that), and he had no fever. There were no abnormal heart sounds; the patient's skin was pink, warm and dry, and the patient was breathing very normally at around 16 breaths per minute. I said that it seemed that all of his vital signs were normal and that there was nothing overtly wrong with him. About that time, the patient said he was fine and that he needed to go to the bathroom. He literally did a 180 degree turnaround – from being seemingly incapacitated to being perfectly fine.

At this point, I was suspecting that the patient might have been putting on somewhat of a show with his symptoms, but I couldn't be sure. I would have reacted in the same matter, even if I had guessed this from the very beginning, since the patient could have really been having a problem.

Immediately after the "event," he informed me that he needed to go to the bathroom.

I wanted the patient to be able to go to the bathroom, but I wanted to make sure that he wasn't going to have another "episode" on his way to the bathroom and end up falling. This was a concern since the patient had reported having severe dizziness. I was NOT going to allow this patient to fall. I suggested that we obtain a urinal for him so that he did not have to walk to the bathroom, but he was totally against it, saying that he felt just fine and wouldn't have a problem getting to the bathroom. However, I insisted that we get a urinal for him, which we ended up doing.

In consulting with my professor afterward, she explained to me that she had several instances such as this one in the past with patients, especially those diagnosed with BPD. In fact, in talking with some of the nurses after the incident, they informed me that during a previous admission, Mr. Rodriguez had pulled the fire alarm, causing one side of the unit to be evacuated, and later in the week, he had claimed that several of the physicians had been coming into his room and telling him that he was a loser. Again, this is just part of the diagnosis, not something the patient really chooses to do, something important for nurses to keep in mind. It's very important not to take these sorts of behaviors personally. The patient does not generally pick out specific staff members that he or she is going to "pick on." It's just who happens to be available at the time.

And that is a lasting message in nursing that I first learned in mental health. Patients may frequently express their emotions in ways that could be taken personally by the nurse. However, in most cases, the anger and/or aggression is not personal. Patients and family members are just reacting to their situation, and sometimes it is related to the patient's disease process.

Ch. 11:
Changing Units

After my time on the general side, I moved to the more intensive side of the unit.

Li Jin was in her 50s. She stood about 5 feet 6 inches tall and had a smile that seemed to warm everyone who she was around, at least on the staff side. One day earlier, she had been admitted to the acute side of the unit because of her apparent paranoid schizophrenia.

I headed to Ms. Jin's room and, after introducing myself and explaining how long I would be with her that day, I took a seat next to her after her prompting and began talking with her.

"How are you feeling today," I asked.

"Oh, I'm just fine really. They have me in here because they think that I am paranoid, but really I'm not."

"Oh," I said. "What reasoning did they give you for admitting you up here?"

"Well, I've stopped taking my medication because I don't need it." Ms. Jin said. "It's so nice outside. I wish I wasn't in here."

"It must be pretty hard being cooped up in here when you could be outside," I said.

We continued the conversation for a few more minutes, and I took a set of vitals on her, which were all within normal limits. I excused myself and made my way back up to the nurses' station to do my preliminary charting and to talk with my clinical instructor to give her the update. I really did not see what the big deal was. After my interaction with her, she seemed to be in touch with reality. She knew that she had been admitted and why, and she was able to have a conversation without having hallucinations or delusions. But I was young and naive.

"Well, I don't know what to tell you, Dr. Keller. She doesn't seem to be too paranoid to me," I said.

"Well keep talking with her. Keep asking some questions and see if everything adds up and makes sense. Most of the time, things aren't quite what they seem," Dr. Keller quipped. She then gave me the grin that only she could give indicating that there was indeed something more going on and that she expected me to realize it pretty soon.

So, back to work I went. Ms. Jin wanted to take a short nap, so I had agreed to come back in about 30 minutes. In the mean time, I worked on charting and looked up a couple more of her medications in depth.

When I made my way back down to her room, I continued to ever-so-gently pry into Ms. Jin's thought process.

"When I was in here earlier, you said that you hadn't been taking your medication. Could you tell me more about that?" I asked.

"Well, I know that I'm supposed to take it, but it makes me feel bad, and I just know that Dr. Lindstrom is out to get me and is in cahoots with my pharmacist and is trying to poison me."

"What makes you suspicious about Dr. Lindstrom and your pharmacist, Ms. Jin?" I asked. I wouldn't have to ask many more questions; all I had to do was nod my head and say "mmhm," as Ms. Jin then went into a very long explanation of her present situation.

"You see, it started several years ago. Dr. Lindstrom took me on as a patient after I had heard some voices one night. I'm convinced they were actually aliens, but my daughters both just knew that I was crazy, so to make them happy I agreed to go to see my physician. Dr. Lindstrom had the hots for me from the beginning. He asked me so many questions about my personal life, and I know that he wanted to get intimate. When I didn't make any moves on him, he prescribed me medication, and when I didn't take it, he had me admitted to the hospital. The aliens just kept coming, though."

"Aha," I thought. "There we go. There was more to the story."

Ms. Jin continued, "He would have his spies come check on me from time to time. He would even send people to my house to set my shrubs on fire and to ring my doorbell and then run off. Men in purple suits would sit in their vehicle just down the street and watch me. I couldn't even go outside. I called 9-1-1 several times, but they eventually wouldn't listen to me anymore because Dr. Lindstrom paid them off."

Her explanation went on for another ten minutes or so. What was so sad yet fascinating about Ms. Jin was that she wholeheartedly believed what she was saying. This was not a story made up by a small child – not an embellishment. No, Ms. Jin truly believed people were out to get her. What then began to occur to me was how terrifying it must be. How would I feel if I truly believed that people were continually out to get me? What would it be like to think that people were watching me at my every turn? How upsetting and terrifying her life must be.

When I went back to the nurses' station the second time, I found Dr. Keller talking with another student, and when I walked into the room, she glanced up at me.

"You were right," I said while shaking my head.

That's all I had to say. She smiled and nodded her head. Later, I explained to her what all I had learned about Ms. Jin. I also told my story to the rest of my clinical group in post-conference as a lesson to all of them that we cannot be too brief and shallow in our assessment of patients.

Ms. Jin taught me that sometimes – no, all of the time – it takes more than a question or two to assess a person's thought process and cognition. There can be a *lot* that does not come out in superficial conversation. And, for some reason, her situation also made me reflect on how terrifying it must be to have a diagnosis like schizophrenia, especially a form that causes the belief that people are out to get the patient. After interacting with Ms. Jin, I truly had an even more empathetic attitude toward the patients I was interacting with on the behavioral health unit. While a broken leg or appendicitis might cause one type of pain, these psychobiologic illinesses cause a type of pain that can be even harder to address.

I'm not sure what became of Ms. Jin. When we returned the next week to clinical, she was no longer on the unit. Even though I did not get to have much follow up with her, she definitely taught be a valuable lesson that I have learned ever since interacting with her.

Ch. 12:
"You trust me?"

"Hello, Mr. Davis," I said as I walked up to the portly middle-aged gentleman sitting in the community area of the behavioral health unit. "My name is John, and I'm a nursing student. I'll be working with you this afternoon and evening."

Mr. Tyrone Davis nodded his head and managed a half smile. I could tell he was nervous, though. He was sitting with his head down but quickly glancing around the room, wringing his hands in his lap. He had been admitted to the unit with mania and had bipolar I disorder. According to his nurse, Lainey, he had spent most of his morning pacing up and down the hallway, and this is the first time he had sat in a long while.

"How are you doing this afternoon?" I asked.

"I'm okay. But I think that I'm going to be constipated."

This was not quite the response I was expecting. Most of the patients on the unit, when asked how they were doing, responded with an explanation of their current emotional state – happy, feeling good, upset, and so forth. I wasn't used to hearing of more somatic concerns. However, this seemed to be Mr. Davis's focus.

"What makes you say that?" I asked Mr. Davis. Before, he answered, he stood up, looking a bit nervous. "Would you like to take a walk?" I asked.

I had found that sometimes with patients that are particularly anxious or have a lot of energy, doing the "walk and talk" can help. It seems that the patient is able to let his or her energy out a bit by walking, and then he or she can focus on the conversation with the nurse more effectively, instead of sitting still the entire time, focusing on their high-energy.

"Yes. Yes," he said. We began pacing up and down the hallway. "Well, my medicine. I think it might be constipating me. And I'm not taking my medicine like I should. I normally take my constipation pills [laxatives] twice a day, but here, they have me taking them once a day, and I don't think it's working."

"Oh, I said. Have you had a chance to speak with a nurse before about this, or would you like me to look into the issue?"

"I haven't said anything. I don't want to upset anyone."

Mr. Davis was a very nice gentleman, and I felt sorry for him. In reading his history in the chart, it was apparent that he had been suffering for well over 20 years with his psychobiologic illness and had several admissions to the hospital. Still, he tried to live as normal a life as he could, with a wife and child and a labor job. He did an outstanding job, really. He took his medicine exactly as prescribed and had his blood levels of lithium drawn exactly as he was told. From the provider perspective, he was an ideal patient. His main problem was that he had begun cycling more rapidly between his deep depression and manic episodes in the previous year or so. Prior to that, he had been well-controlled. His psychiatrist had tried several different combinations of medications, but nothing seemed to be helping.

After our discussion about the constipation and doing a physical assessment on Mr. Davis, I went to find Lainey so that I could tell her of Mr. Davis's concern. I really respected Lainey because she was the true epitome of patient advocate, and she was very nice to nursing students. She was only in her mid-twenties and had not been a nurse for too long, so I think she remembered what it was like to be a student – unsure and sometimes scared to ask questions. I knew I could approach her with any question or comment, and I also knew that she would do all she could to help her patients.

I found Lainey preparing an injection near the medicine cart. "Hi," she said with a smile.

"Hi, Lainey. You know Mr. Davis, right?" I asked.

"Yep. How's he doing? Still anxious and full of energy?"

"Well, he definitely has energy still. We just spent about 10 minutes walking the hallway," I commented.

"Oh yeah. I saw you guys walking. It looked like he was talking quite a bit," she noted.

"He is very concerned about his constipation and especially his laxative," I explained. "When he is at home, he says that he takes it twice a day, but when he was admitted, they changed it to once per day, but it's the same total dosage."

"Hmm," Lainey replied. "Let's give Dr. Riley a call and see if we can split that up to twice a day. If Mr. Davis says it helped to have it in a split dose, then we should believe him."

"I'm on board with that," I replied.

This is why I really liked Lainey. She recognized that patients know their bodies best, even when they might be admitted to the behavioral health unit. Sure, there are those times when patients are totally disconnected from reality, but they still have important contributions they can make to their care. She respected patients' opinions and feelings, and this was an example of that.

While Lainey dialed Dr. Riley to see about changing the medication, I made my way back down the short hallway to Mr. Davis's room. There, I found him wringing his hands again, while sitting on the edge of his bed. There was another male in the room now – a visitor.

"Oh, hello," I said. "I'm John, a student nurse."

"Hi, I'm Tyrone's nephew, Marcus Daniels," he replied. "Tyrone says you are trying to help him with his constipation right now."

"That's right, I said. I've talked with Lainey, and she is contacting Dr. Riley as we speak to see if we can get that laxative dose split up to twice per day."

Mr. Davis seemed pleased with this response, though he still looked nervous. About that time, the intercom kicked on, and Betty, the unit clerk, announced that supper had arrived. This meant that patients could go to the common area to eat their meal. I could tell Mr. Davis was ready to eat his food, so I decided to go back to the nurses' station and let Mr. Davis enjoy his meal. "Anything else I can do for you right now, Mr. Davis?" I asked.

"No," he responded. "I think I'll go eat now."

As Mr. Davis walked out, his nephew, Marcus, stopped me and wanted to talk.

"Do you have a second?" Mr. Daniels asked me.

"Sure," I said. "What would you like to discuss?"

"Well, Tyrone has always been like a dad to me, since my daddy left my mom and me when I was young, and I just want what is best for him. He thinks that his new bipolar medicine is causing his side effects. What do you think? If you think it might be causing it, could we talk to the physican about changing it?"

This question took me back. It was happening again. Just like that time in my introductory nursing course, a family member was asking *me* for my opinion – my "expert" opinion.

"What in the world," I thought. "He wants to know what *I* think? But I'm just a nursing student. How could he trust me? I'm not a pharmacist. I'm not an expert in psychiatric medications. Are these people out of their minds?"

I answered honestly and said that I wasn't sure but that I would check for him, which I did. There was no mention of constipation in the drug reference system, and I couldn't even find any case reports of constipation caused by the drug, which I cannot even remember the name of now.

As the rest of the evening progressed, I began reflecting on what had transpired. I began to realize how trusted nurses are. Sure, we had been told in lecture that nurses are one of the most, if not the most, trusted professions, but it was different experiencing this trust.

Indeed, it was a small piece of trust, simply asking about a medication, but this nephew had enough confidence in me to trust me with answering a question about his beloved uncle's health, and that meant a lot. I felt so unsure of myself internally, but externally, I guess I was able to seem knowledgable and trustworthy.

After this day, I would be asked my opinion about things more and more by patients and family members, and even nurses began asking me what my interpretation of a lab result was or what I had found in my assessment. However, my day with Mr. Davis was really the beginning of the realization that nurses are special and have a special relationship with patients and their families, and the trust that is shown and absolutely necessary in nursing should never be broken.

As it turned out, the dosing of the laxative had been an oversight, and Dr. Riley was fine with Mr. Davis taking his medication twice a day instead of once daily. When I told him about it, Mr. Davis was ecstatic. This relatively small detail, the dosing of his laxative, had been nagging at him since his admission, and by advocating for the patient in such a small way, it made a world of difference. From that point on, Mr. Davis seemed more relaxed and did not seem as preoccupied. While he was still in his manic phase, psychologically, he was so much more relaxed. Sometimes, actually a lot of times, it is the small things in a patient's life that matter, and by addressing these, we can help make the patient experience better and improve quality of life.

Ch. 13:
Stress and Anxiety, Part 1

While my time in clinical was always fairly unpredictable and allowed me to work with patients and hone my clinical skills, life outside of clinical was much more predictable, tedious and, most of the time, stressful. Once I returned home from clinical, the world did not stop and simply allow me to complete all of the post-clinical work I needed to accomplish, just as the world never really stops for anyone, any time.

At this point in my academic career, I had a lot of irons in the fire – not only was I a busy student with 18 credit hours, but I was working as a tutor for the Writing Center and also for the Office of Student Success. This meant spending several hours each week tutoring and attending staff meetings. I cannot really complain, though, as tutoring was one of my favorite times during the week, and it is really what reinforced the idea that I wanted to be a nurse educator some day. In addition to tutoring, I sat on the School of Nursing Curriculum Committee, and I would soon be serving as a senator on the Student Senate, so I had quite a few meetings to attend. As if this were not enough, I was also working on a research project with my advisor and another student, which took up several more hours per week. Of course, looking back, I wouldn't have changed any of this involvement, as it is what made my undergraduate years fantastic. My research allowed me to present research across the United States in places like Chicago, Louisville, Kentucky, and St. Joseph, Missouri. Additionally, I was able to publish an academic journal article in the *Journal of Psychosocial Nursing and Mental Health Services.*

While I was, externally, able to balance and handle all of these responsibilities, internally, it was much more difficult. My peers, professors and family all seemed to have the same attitude.

"Oh, you've always been able to balance all kinds of things, so you'll be able to do that this semester, too," they would say.

But I was not so sure. My anxieties about clinical – whether I would "mess up" or accidentally do something I shouldn't – were ever-present, and I put a lot of extra pressure on myself, aiming for straight As. This pressure was not really present from my family; rather, it was something that I had self-induced on myself. While there are those students constantly bombarded by their parents' tirades about studying and being on the Dean's list, my parents were much more relaxed, probably because they knew I had good self-discipline and would govern my own studying habits. They frequently encouraged me to enjoy college more and not worry as much about classes – especially those not directly related to nursing.

It was hard for me, though. I always wanted to do my best because, well, I would have patients' lives in my hands, and I didn't want to miss something I should have learned during school that could cost a patient in the future. I knew that I couldn't know everything – it was impossible, after all. However, my goal was to learn as much as humanly possible.

What's more, nursing exams were just getting harder and harder and causing more anxiety. Without taking one of these exams, it is pretty hard to explain what makes them difficult. In short, many questions come with several answers that could be correct, but there is one "best" answer. For example, a question might ask the student to select the "best therapeutic response to the patient." The choices would include four items that a nurse could legitimately say to a patient, but one of them would be the "most correct." This kind of question was a nuisance to me and the rest of my nursing cohort, and I'm sure any nursing students or nurses reading this can empathize with me.

Another sort of question that would consistently nag at us was the "multiple response" question. For these questions, we would have to select all answers that applied. Therefore, if given five answer choices, all five could be correct or none of them could be correct. Perhaps the first two and the last choice were correct but not the third and fourth. It never failed that I would get all but one correct. I would circle A and B but not circle D, even though it was correct, or I would circle four out of five, and it turned out that all five choices were correct. This left me with no credit for the question, however, since these were all-or-nothing questions – no partial credit, unfortunately.

With every exam I walked into, it felt like my stomach was in my throat, and my pulse would always go up 15 or 20 beats per minute. I wasn't alone, either; several of my classmates ended up on anti-anxiety and anti-depressant medication during our nursing school tenure.

This stress ended up manifesting itself a couple times, which scared me into addressing my stress. On one occasion, I was at a family party enjoying myself and talking with several people in the driveway. There were at least 15 people there that day. A family friend asked me, "How's school going?"

"It's pretty stressful," I responded. "I've got a lot of credits plus clinical and extra-curricular stuff, and there's not a lot of time to enjoy myself."

"Ha! That's nothing," he said. "Just wait until you get to the real world."

And at that moment, I exploded. "What do you mean, you insane man? When I *get* to the real world," I was thinking. What I said was not much better.

"Why don't you, sir, come to my world and live a few weeks under the stressors I put up with, and then you can tell me that my stress is nothing." I really let him have it. "You think your life is so stressful, and if it is, okay, but that doesn't mean that my life is not stressful! You don't even know my life!"

At that moment, I realized that my outburst was uncalled for. I think my frontal cortex finally caught up to the emotional centers in my brain and instructed me to back off and go take a breather, which I did.

I ended up reflecting on this incident many times. What had caused me to lash out in the way I had? Sure, I had been slightly provoked, but this was so very uncharacteristic of me. I always a reserved, non-confrontational person, and to yell at a grown adult in the middle of a family party was unheard of. I always tried to listen to others and critically reflect on what they said before I responded, and in this case, I was jumping to a response irrationally.

I decided that it was time for a change. I had to let myself enjoy life a little more, or I would have more of these outbursts, I was sure. The stress was really getting to me, and it was becoming evident. I knew that I was, internally, suffering from the stress and anxiety – having problems sleeping and worrying about just about everything, but now it was beginning to show itself externally. Luckily, the semester was almost over at this point, and I would have a chance to re-charge before the next semester and could also choose to do more for myself in the coming semesters.

I decided to include this chapter, as I know there are a lot of nursing students in a situation similar to mine. Heck, I didn't even have a spouse, children or other life-concerns of that nature. I knew several students during my time in school with a husband and children at home, car payments, and house payments. I give them the utmost respect; how did they do it?

The message here is that we all need to find time to re-energize ourselves. We cannot be perfect 100% of the time. Whether it's taking an hour out of the day to just lie on a bed and listen to music, enjoying a nice warm shower, or taking half a day to enjoy time with friends, it's important to make the time. I know it's not always possible to take this time, and sometimes we do have to delay gratification, especially in nursing school, but more times than not, I think it's important to strive for these time-outs when it is possible to recharge. The human body can only endure so much continual stress before it breaks down.

PART III: Maternal-Child Nursing

Maternal-child nursing, commonly called "peds/OB," was a totally different world. Pediatrics was certainly not my cup of tea, but as it turned out, OB was almost a second calling.

Ch. 14:
Welcome to Peds/OB

"We're going to be getting a 10 week old baby boy with a skull fracture," said Danielle, the RN I was working with in the pediatric special care unit. "We don't know much else though until the ER calls up to give us more information."

There aren't a lot of ways a baby can "accidentally" get a skull fracture. In general, 10 week olds aren't active enough on their own to accomplish such an injury. Many times when a baby this age has a skull fracture, it stems from physical abuse, which was our main concern.

"Of course," I thought. "My first day on pediatrics and I'm dealing with an abuse case."

We waited for about 15 minutes for the ER to call, and when they did, we found out that the story was not quite as ominous as we had first thought. As Danielle received the report from the ER nurse, I anxiously waited, trying to read her face in order to get an indication of what was going on. After she got off the phone, Danielle let out a "happy sigh" and cracked a half smile.

"Apparently, the mother of this little boy had been making breakfast for her other children and had the baby swaddled up in a thick blanket. She was holding on to the bottom of the blanket and thought she had a hold of her son's legs, but, in fact, she only had a good hold on the lower portion of the thick blanket. She leaned a little bit too much when reaching for something, and the baby spiraled out of the blanket and fell approximately 4 feet to the floor," Danielle said. "I'm sure glad this doesn't sound like an abuse case. Of course, we will have to be very cautious and be sure to assess for any suspicious behaviors of the family and make sure that there is indeed no abuse going on," she added.

Before the baby was brought up to the floor, the ER physician wanted to get a full skeletal study of the baby, just to be sure there were no other injuries. This study is no small feat, however. It involves taking x-rays of all of the major bones in the body, including the arms, legs, hands, feet, chest, and so forth. I went downstairs so that I could help with this series of x-rays, as it takes several people to keep a 10 week old still. In fact, though it almost seemed like torture, in order to get a good x-ray of the baby's hand, the hand had to be taped down to the x-ray plate. By some miracle, the only injury this baby suffered was a small skull fracture.

Once the baby made it up to the floor, Danielle and I performed a full head-to-toe assessment on the baby and assessed vital signs, which were all normal. The baby had a nice, lusty cry and had all normal reflexes intact. The only evidence of injury was the great big bruise on his head and a swollen eye.

In the end, we ended up providing almost more care to the parents – especially the mother. She was beside herself that she had actually caused a skull fracture in her child. "Never will I ever do anything else when I'm holding him," she said in an exasperated voice.

While I was excited to start another semester of nursing school, I wasn't sure how things would go, considering working with children was not quite my forte. And, indeed this first day presented me with the unique challenge of dealing with a very small, delicate patient.

Ch. 15:
Jacob

Sometimes we needed to be reminded of how lucky we really are, especially when we think our life is pretty stressful.

Jacob Shields was in the home-stretch of his freshman year of college. He was an intelligent, 19-year-old student who had managed a solid GPA and several co-curricular activities during his first year of college away in Missouri. A few weeks before spring break, Jacob, during one of his routine weekly calls with his mother, Debbie, had noted that he had become increasingly fatigued and that he was beginning to notice difficulty paying attention in class. He described it as "just not feeling right." His mother didn't think much of it at the time, chalking it up to a 19-year-old in college who probably wasn't getting the amount of sleep he should and probably not taking care of his body as well as he could.

When Jacob returned home for spring break, though, he just didn't seem right. When he arrived home, he said hello to his mother, father and sister but then layed down on the couch and fell asleep. He stayed asleep for several hours before his mother woke him for supper. He immediately went back to bed after eating, though. When he woke up in the morning, he noted that he had experienced a nosebleed overnight. He felt like he had a little more energy, but it only came in short bursts, and then he was back to feeling exhausted.

Later in the day, he was playing with his dog Sam, a golden retriever. Sam had jumped up on the couch with Jacob and was walking all over his legs, trying to find a good place to sit with Jacob on the couch. He did, and the two spent time on the couch together, until Jacob fell asleep. At supper time, Jake noticed dark purple spots on his legs and couldn't figure out what they were. However, as the evening progressed, they began to obviously present themselves as bruises. And there weren't just a couple of them. All over both of his legs, on the top side, were bruises. This made no sense. Sure, Sam the dog had been walking on Jacob's legs, but there was no reason for brusies to have formed.

When Debbie learned of the significant brusising, she told Jacob that he needed to go see a doctor immediately. She drove him to one of the express clinics in town, and the nurse practitioner there was quite concerned about Jacob, given his physical symptoms. She ordered several laboratory tests, including a complete blood count. When the results of this test came back, they had their answer. Jacob's white blood cell count was 76,000, which is very, very high for a young male who should have a count somewhere between 4,500 and 10,500 (depending on the laboratory).

Becaue of Jacob's extreme fatigue at this point, he was admitted to the hospital in which I was doing my clinical rotation. After reviewing the blood samples under a microscope, it was determined that Jacob had leukemia. At the hospital, he was transferred from the general medical unit to the pediatrics unit so that he could be seen by a pediatric oncologist, since the type of cancer he had, acute lymphocytic leukemia, is very common in children, and these pediatric oncologists are used to dealing with this type of cancer.

I did not have a lot of interaction with Jacob, as he was not my patient for the day; he was actually being taken care of by one of my classmates, Shelly. However, Jacob and his family told Shelly Jacob's story, and in a relatively tearful post-conference, Shelly told us the story. Because it was still early on in his diagnosis, there was no certainty as to the prognosis. His oncologist was going to start chemotherapy immediately, but it would take a while to see how well this treatment approach was going to work. Indeed, Jacob would be in for a lot, and it was highly unlikely that he would be able to finish out his second semester of college.

Reflecting on this experience, I think all of us realized just how lucky we actually were (and are). At the time in the semester that we encountered Jacob, we were all stressed out, worrying about upcoming exams, finishing lengthy papers and working on taxing care plans. There was not a lot of time for relaxation and fun. However, after being faced with the reality that our lives could be so much worse, we all had a better perspective, and I think it put us in our places, so to speak.

Ch. 16:
Love Makes a Difference

For this clinical experience, the only information I had came via email. We were to be given our patient's diagnosis and age but no other information, so I logged into my email account and opened the email from Professor Davidson. "John – 6 mo. old male; hemangioma & tethered spinal cord; propranolol trial."

Well, I had two things going for me. I knew what a hemangioma was, since we had studied skin lesions in health assessment the previous semester. However, I had no idea what really causes the lesions. Second, I knew what propranolol is – a beta blocker medication that lowers heart rate and blood pressure. As for a tethered spinal cord, I was, for all intents and purposes, clueless. Sure, I had an idea that this diagnosis was related to the spinal cord and somehow involved tethering, but I was grossly unaware of the technical aspects of this diagnosis. This meant a few hours of studying; to the library I went.

As I found out, hemangiomas (also called strawberry lesions or strawberry marks) are collections of blood vessels that are abnormal and are present on the skin. Many times, these look like strawberries because they present as bright red bumps or masses. The more superficial strawberry hemangiomas are generally benign, exist before birth, and continue to grow as a baby gets older – up to around one year – while the deeper hemangiomas may be more severe and could result in problems with organs, especially if blood flow is significantly impacted. If the hemangioma is located in pressure-sensitive areas, such as the spinal cord, pressure could be increased as the hemangioma grows, leading to other functional problems. Beta blocker medications, and specifically propranolol, may help cause a large angioma to "shrink" or resolve from its protruding appearance to flat or almost flat. This was the primary reason that this child had been admitted to the hospital – to monitor the infant's blood pressure and heart rate.

Hemangiomas may be signs of more serious problems, however. Hemangiomas that occur in the lower back area of newborns need to be investigated further, as they may indicate a significant underlying abnormality, even in children that present with a normal neurologic exam, as was the case with my patient.

Aside from the hemangioma, the more serious problem, a tethered spinal cord, is a spinal cord that is attached by tissue somewhere along the spinal column (bones or other tissues) that it is not supposed to be attached, causing pulling and stretching. This attachment can occur at various points along the spinal column. This condition is related to spina bifida, as both problems originate from the neural tube during fetal development and an improper separation of the spinal cord and surrounding tissue.

While the initial issue of tissue attachment itself might not be a major issue, the problems arise as the patient begins to grow. As the person grows, the spinal cord must adapt with this growth, rising upward through the spinal column as the person's length increases. In normal fetal development, the spinal cord starts out at the very base of the spinal column in the sacral area, but the spinal cord does not grow as fast as the rest of the body and also ends up being shorter than the spinal column itself. If the spinal cord is attached to the sides or base of the spinal column, as the surrounding tissues continue to grow and the human begins to grow in length, the spinal cord needs to be able to ascend through the spinal column; however, when the spinal cord is inadvertently attached to the surrounding tissue at some point, as in a tethered spinal cord, the spinal cord is not able to move, and stretching occurs. As the person grows more and more, certain neurological problems begin to present. For example, pain in the legs or back and numbness in the feet may be one of the first signs, followed by a difficulty in walking and bowel/urinary incontinence.

Because of the problems a tethered spinal cord can have over time, treatment is needed, and the earlier the better, as problems can be avoided if the spinal cord (and rest of the spinal column) is allowed to develop normally as the person matures. Surgery is the only treatment that will cure the condition, and the invasiveness of the surgery varies significantly, based on where the tethering is located and how much of the spinal cord and surrounding tissue is involved. Luckily, these surgeries generally go smoothly, and children are allowed to develop normally. The prognosis for this condition is good, and life expectancy is the same as the general population.

After several hours of preparation, the clock read 10:35 PM, and I decided it was time to head to bed so that I could wake up at 5:45 AM the next morning. Sure enough, the hours ticked by more quickly than I wanted, and my cell phone's alarm clock so annoyingly began to ring at 5:45 AM on the dot. Oh, how I longed to be able to push the "snooze" button several times. But, alas, I needed to head to the shower. And, so, as always, I began my morning half-awake, half-zombie routine.

In the early morning hours, my eyes tended to be open just enough to (unsuccessfully, I might add) prevent myself from running into something as I maneuvered around . . . bumping into the wall here, running into the counter there. At times I felt like a toddler just learning to walk, the only thing propelling me forward being the inertia of my very first step I took after getting up out of bed.

On this morning, I decided I would brush my teeth first, so I turned the water on to prepare to wet my toothbrush and picked up a round tube – what I thought was toothpaste. After pre-rinsing my toothbrush, a habit I have always had, I squeezed a one-inch ribbon of "toothpaste" onto my toothbrush and inserted the utensil into my mouth.

But it wasn't toothpaste.

In my comatose-like morning state, I had actually reached for one of my roommate's items; I enjoyed a nice mouthful of "Pure Romance" shaving cream. I wasn't feeling very romantic. After spitting and washing my mouth out repeatedly, I remember shaking my head and asking, "Who puts shaving cream in tubes?" in a rather exasperated tone. What a wake-up call that had been. "Let's hope the day starts going better," I noted.

Once I finally made it to the hospital, I needed to find out more information on my patient. Since we only received a limited amount of information prior to the clinical day, I had to get to the hospital a bit earlier to facilitate this information collection. My patient that day was Conner Cade Cooper, a whole six months old. "What alliteration in his name," I thought to myself. "His parents must have had a literary sense about them."

Indeed, as I had been tipped off to the night before, Conner had been admitted for a propranolol trial to try to reduce the size of his hemangioma prior to surgery for his tethered spinal cord. At this point, he was a normally functioning child, given that his length had not increased enough for his spinal cord to be stretched. While he was in the hospital, we would be primarily concerned with monitoring his vital signs to make sure that the medication did not depress his blood pressure or heart rate too much. This would be the "easy" part of the day, however.

What I have neglected to mention was that my pediatrics rotation had put about as much fear in me as my psychiatric-mental health rotation had. As an only child with a fairly small immediate family and not many younger cousins, I had only held one baby in my lifetime up to that point – my cousin Katie. However, at the time, I was only 12 years old, and I was sitting on a couch with a pillow on my lap, hoping for dear life that I didn't drop her.

That was about the extent of the interactions I had with babies. I had never changed a diaper; never held a baby while standing; never rocked a baby to sleep; never fed a baby with a bottle; never negotiated the placement of a pacifier into a screaming mouth. However, this day, I would do all of these things. This would be the real challenge. While I still felt like a rookie nursing student, I felt even more like a rookie dealing with babies.

I would somehow have to convince his parents to allow me to care for him, even though I had essentially no experience working with babies. "How would I feel if a nursing student came in and wanted to take care of my pride and joy?" I had wondered. As it turned out, Conner's mom Deidra was more than happy to allow me to work with Conner. In fact, she even helped me as I blundered several feats.

Conner was a sweet baby, I had to admit. He looked up from his crib, smiling, reaching with his hands for something he saw but not within his grasp. His little chubby legs and cheeks were too lovable not to notice. But what was also noticeable was the smell of a dirty diaper. "Oh, terrific," I noted begrudgingly. "Here goes nothing . . ."

There were already diapers in the room, ready to be applied to the baby's bottom. But how did they work? I opened up one of the diapers and set it in the hospital crib and then began to take off the dirty diaper. This seemed simple enough, and it was. But then came wiping his bottom. I had baby wipes available, and used them readily, but with each wipe there was more to wipe. About 10 wipes later, and I still couldn't seem to get his bottom clean. As I found out, the problem was that I wasn't using enough force; I was being too gentle in my wiping, afraid I would somehow damage Conner. Deidra stepped in to help.

After the wiping came the application of the new diaper. This would prove to be the peace de résistance – or not. I picked up the new diaper and held it up in the air, closely examining it like a unidentified flying object. Now what? What end went under the buttocks? Which tab went to the font and which to the back? What did this blue line running down the length of the diaper mean? I was in trouble. I began foolishly trying to maneuver the diaper under Conner, as he giggled uncontrollably – I'm convinced secretly mocking me, though I did find it pretty adorable. Deidra saw me struggling and walked over to offer her assistance – again. She didn't talk down to me and actually took the moment to walk me through each step, though. I admitted that I had never actually changed a diaper, and she understood, not overtly passing judgment on me.

Later in the day, I fed Conner. Deidra and Conner's father, Donald, had both left for about an hour to get some lunch themselves, so I had Conner "all to myself." This was actually the first time they had left Conner's side in about 24 hours, so it was a big deal to them. I could tell Conner had so much love surrounding him.

Feeding was a challenge, too. How was I to maneuver Conner and hold the bottle and also keep him from eating too quickly? He had a one-inch diameter hemangioma on his lower back after all. How would I hold him in a way that wouldn't disrupt this lesion?

He loved his bottle, as I found out, and he rarely came up for air. After feeding him, the frightening reality hit me that I would need to burp him. After all, he had inhaled the bottle and undoubtedly copious amounts of air. I actually had to *hold* him – this small, delicate, easily injured tiny human. This called for backup.

I left Conner in his crib for a minute and went out to the desk to find a fellow nursing student more qualified in matters of this nature. I located Molly, who had several younger siblings and who had also helped care for those siblings. She teased me the entire time as she walked me through the proper way to hold Conner to most effectively facilitate patting on his back to help built-up air escape his bloated belly. He seemed happy enough with my performance, but the entire time I was holding him and burping him, I was terrified. I thought I might drop him. I thought I might accidentally disturb his hemangioma. I thought he might vomit on me. I thought he might start screaming. Basically, I imagined the worst possible scenario.

After burping him, I placed him supine in the crib, but he began to cry and scream, looking around, seemingly searching for his parents. "Oh jeez. Oh jeez," I though. I reached for a pacifier in the room, hoping to pacify him. He wouldn't take it. I repeatedly tried to insert the small device in his mouth, but I was unsuccessful. Why wouldn't he take it? About that time, Professor Davidson walked in and chuckled a bit.

"Having trouble getting him to settle down?" she asked me.

"Uh… Yeah," I responded. "Any ideas? I've tried the pacifier, but he won't take it."

"Here, let me try," she answered. "Sometimes you have to make a game out of it."

She then started making funny faces at Conner and made the pacifier fly like a Boeing 747 on approach to the runway. "Here comes the plane Conner. Here it comes," she said in a "baby" voice.

Sure enough, it worked. Conner seemed transfixed by Professor Davidson. She had done it. Something I had attempted for about five minutes. All it took as a game and some funny faces.

The rest of the day went well, and I was able to complete my charting in an efficient manner. Conner would be discharged the next morning, provided his vital signs all remained stable. So far, the medication had not caused any significant issues, only dropping his heart rate slightly and dropping his blood pressure about 10 to 15 millimeters of mercury (the unit of measure in which blood pressure is taken). Surgery would be scheduled fairly soon, once the hemangioma had a little time to shrink.

In post-conference, I told the stories from the day – including my blunders and befuddled attempts. My classmates got a good laugh at my expense, but that was okay. None of us were perfect, and we all knew we had a lot to learn, even if the learning was very basic.

What I also heard about in post-conference was how different one of my classmates' days had gone. While I was working with a family that shared a lot of love, Chelle had worked with a baby who had been admitted with several suspicious bone fractures, as well as many bruises. In fact, the Department of Children and Family Services (DCFS) had been called in to investigate, and Chelle had spent several hours of her day dealing with parents that had apparently taken their aggression out on their child, though they didn't admit to it. She also took care of the child while DCFS questioned the parents. During our meeting, Chelle tearfully described her encounters that day, and I knew that experience would have a permanent impact on her life, as well as many of us in the room.

"How lucky am I to have a loving family?" I thought to myself. "Even when things aren't going well and I feel like quitting, I've got more going for me than some people. I know I have a support system that will be there for me, and I know I am unconditionally loved. That's more than Chelle's patient could say for himself."

Love does make a difference.

Ch. 17:
"Here comes the baby!"

"If you fail to make sure the baby's identification bracelet matches the person whom you are giving the child to, you will fail clinical – no questions asked." This action could also result in dismissal from the school of nursing altogether.

Dr. Fraley meant business, and she wanted us to know that it was absolutely critical that we keep the babies that would be under our care safe. She also always made it quite clear that we were acting in the role of a nurse, and, as such, patients were *our* responsibility, not anyone else's. I wasn't sure what to expect coming into my obstetrics clinical rotation, but as I found out, it's different than what I imagined, especially being a male. It would also be a thrilling rotation, and, all-in-all, I would see three new lives brought into the world, two by vaginal birth and one by a cesarean section.

I traipsed up the stairs of the back stairwell at the hospital. It was about 6:30 AM, so I was still wiping my eyes to get the blur out, but I knew that this day could be the one that I saw a baby be born. I was assigned to labor and delivery, and since there was no way to know what patient would be in labor the next day, we had prepared a general care plan for a laboring woman and were to be ready for whatever might come our way.

Once I arrived at the labor and delivery unit, I made my way to the small conference room and plopped down in the chair, nervous yet ready to get going. Only one of my clinical classmates, Emma, was there.

"Well, you ready?" she asked.

"Uhh. Good question. I don't know." That was my only response.

Everyone had assembled by just a little before 7:00, and Dr. Fraley came into the room with our assignments in hand.

I was first. "John, you've got a 28-year-old multip. Her name is Hannah Gesell. She's got Pit running at 2 milliunits per minute and had an epidural placed about half an hour ago. So far, things are progressing well, and she's about 3 centimeters, 60% effaced. She has two IV lines, one in the left AC, an 18 guage, and also one in the right AC, a 20 gauge – also has some lactated Ringer's going at 80 milliliters per hour. She's down in room 1822, and apparently her husband is in there with her. Any questions? If not, get going."

Basically, to translate what Dr. Fraley said, this was not the patient's first baby (she was "multiparous" or a "multip"), and she was on an intravenous drip of Pitocin, a drug that is a synthetic version of the body's hormone oxytocin. Oxytocin is a major hormone involved in causing contractions in females during labor. Additionally, the woman was receiving pain relief from the epidural, which is basically like an intravenous line going into the epidural space around the vertebral colum. She wasn't too far along, since she was only 3 centimeters dilated and 60% effaced, but since this was not her first child, it was possible she would progress rather quickly. She also had two intravenous lines in, one delivering some fluids and the other delivering Pitocin.

I didn't have any questions to ask Dr. Fraley, so I got up and pushed my chair in and headed for the door. In reality, I had a lot of questions – but none to ask her. Would I be able to keep my composure during the delivery process? Would I really be able to reassure the mother that I, a *male* nursing student, could help her through the labor process and keep her baby safe? Sure, I had many, many questions but none that I could really ask out loud.

I turned left out of the break room and began the 30 or 40 yard walk down to the nurse's station so that I could do a quick chart check on the patient before I went to the room. The butterflies on the wallpaper were not the only "butterflies" at that moment. My stomach, too, contained its share.

After briefly reviewing the patient's chart, I learned that she had received a full complement of prenatal care, and there were no red flags. All tests and assessments had come back normal, so the hope was that this labor and delivery would be straightforward and uneventful.

Now it was time – time to go to the patient's room. Normally, there was a small amount of anxiety prior to entering the patient's room for the first time; in this case, though, my anxiety level was through the roof. I had no idea what to expect. Would the husband welcome having another male in the room while his wife labored? Would he allow me to perform the necessary assessments on his wife? Would the laboring patient want me to be hands-on with the labor, or would she want me to stay in the corner and not look at anything? Again, so many questions raced through my mind.

I approached the room cautiously. When I made it to the door, I could hear a faint sound of music. This would end up being the patient's own radio that she had brought with her in order to make the labor process just a bit more pleasant. No lights were on in the room, and I hoped I wouldn't be waking up the patient or her husband. I knocked a few times on the door, and the patient said, "yes?"

This was my big moment. How I presented myself and the first impression I made with the patient and her husband would likely dictate how willing they would be to allow me into their very special moment in time.

"Hi," I said. "My name is John, and I'm a nursing student from Millikin University doing my labor and delivery roation right now."

"Hello," Mrs. Gesell said smiling. Her husband had been napping, and he smiled, half-awake. I had a feeling she knew what was coming.

It seemed like my first impression was going well enough, since both parties were at least smiling. Still, I decided I needed to legitimize myself, since I was "only" a student, so I also said, "If it's alright with you, I'd like to work with you during your labor and delivery. You would be my only patient, so I'd be able to closely watch the fetal monitor and keep an eye on all of your medications and monitors." I hoped that by showing them the potential benefit of having a student dedicated to the patient and her unborn baby, she and her husband would be more willing to allow me in.

Apparently, it worked. Both she and her husband were more than happy to have me in the room. Once I had permission to enter, I got to work.

I first started with some baseline vital signs, taking a look at the patient's last blood pressure, and pressing the button so that the machine would take another pressure. I counted the mom's respirations and checked her pulse, both of which were normal. And, finally, I took Mrs. Gesell's temperature. Her "water" (amniotic sac) broke about an hour before I had arrived, so she was at an increased risk of infection, since bacteria could potentially make its way up the vaginal canal and into the cervix and uterus, especially after people started doing vaginal exams to check on the progress of the baby. I checked the IV flow rate, along with the Pitocin and epidural. Everything in the infusion department looked good, thank goodness.

I then focused my attention on the baby, whose "whoosh, whoosh, whoosh" heartbeat could be heard from the ultrasound machine. I looked at the electronic fetal monitoring (EFM) unit sitting next to the mom's bed, which displayed not only the calculated fetal heart rate but also the mother's last blood pressure, current heart rate, and contraction occurances in wave form. To obtain the EFM, two straps with disc-looking objects are placed around the mother's abdomen. One of these discs reveals the baby's heart rate, and the other helps to show when the mom is having a contraction (called the tocodynamometer, which is perhaps one of the coolest words to say in nursing).

When monitoring is being done from the outside, the tocodynamometer, also known affectionately as the "toco," shows when the uterus is contracting, as it is more compressed by the abdomen during a contraction. However, the arches that show upon the screen demonstrating a contraction do not really reveal exactly how strong a contraction is, since there are some variables that could impact the true strength. (If internal monitoring is implemented, a catheter with a pressure device can actually be inserted into the uterus, and, in this case, contraction strength can be measured more accurately.) Since the toco in external monitoring is not able to tell the strength of contractions, I had to be sure to manually palpate (feel) the mother's abdomen from the start to the end of the contraction to estimate the strength of the contraction. I was sure to check not only how strong the contractions were but also how long they were lasting and how far apart they were ocurring, which at that point was about every 3 to 4 minutes. The baby's heart was still beating away at around 150 beats per minute, nice and strong.

As a last step in my initial assessment, I pulled out the eight-foot-long length of paper that had printed from the EFM. The entire time the patient is hooked up to the EFM machine, this machine prints out, fairly slowly, a tracing showing the baby's heart rate, the mother's contractions, and any other vital signs that are taken by the machine or recorded by the nurse. It was important to make sure that the baby's heart rate was remaining stable and that contractions were progressing nicely. This historical assessment is quite important. Even though the EFM machine gives a current report, the baseline data is what I was really after at this point, especially in regard to the baby. For example, even if the baby's heart rate were 130, which is considered normal, if I looked at the long strip of paper summarizing the baby's heart rate for the last four hours and noticed that for a solid three hours the heart rate had been in the 150s and had slowly been decreasing over the last hour, that would tell me something might be going on that needs to be addressed. At this point in my assessment, though, all was well; the baby's heart rate had been varying nicely the entire time from between the 140s and the 150s. It just seemed too good to be true; mom and baby were doing just fine, and all was right with the world.

About that time, Dr. Fraley walked in the room and requested that I "tell me [her] about the patient." In not-so-many words, this meant that I was to give her a run-down of everything that I had assessed and what my plan was for this patient moving forward. Of course, being a clinical instructor, her job was to make me think and also to ensure that I was providing safe care. As such, it was almost impossible to please Dr. Fraley 100%. I could cover 95% of the material she wanted me to, but not reporting just one important piece of assessment data could cause a stern correction to come my way.

While I felt more comfortable with clinical instructors that were a bit more "gentle" in their approach, having a clinical instructor that gave us a swift kick in the rear when we needed it was also appreciated. In Dr. Fraley's case, she certainly made sure we realized the magnitude of our role as not only a student nurse but as a nurse in general. While the common misconception is that nursing students practice solely under their instructor's license and aren't held liable for things gone wrong during clinical, in fact, students are just as liable as their instructors. Dr. Fraley made sure we understood that. She also wanted us to realize that small errors can actually result in serious complications later.

Indeed, I covered everything she wanted me to – except one item. I had not yet checked to see if the mother planned to breast feed or bottle feed after the baby was born. "Well how do you expect the baby to attach to the mom immediately after birth, if she is planning on breast feeding," Dr. Fraley asked me. "Uh, well . . . good question," I responded.

In my mind, this was not a huge deal. I wouldn't be delivering the baby, after all, and there would be "actual" nurses in the room with the patient who knew what to do after the baby was born. Nonetheless, I would never again forget to ask the mother what nutrition option she was going to select for her baby.

Mrs. Gesell's labor progressed very rapidly as the morning progressed. Dr. Fraley left the room around 8:00 AM, and Mrs. Gesell was ready to push at 10:00 AM. "I just feel like I need to push," she had told me. "It feels like I'm full and have to get the baby out!"

I had the job of holding the left leg, while the labor nurse held her right leg back. Every time Mrs. Gesell was to push, the labor nurse and I would push the patient's legs back and out a little bit to help with the labor progress. In this case, Mrs. Gesell only had to push about ten times before a healthy baby girl was delivered.

Seeing a baby delivered was, without a doubt, one of the most memorable moments of nursing school. While it was quite graphic and involved a lot of bodily fluids, the ability to be present when a new life was brought into the world was a great privilege and very much worth it.

And, by some miracle, the husband didn't question my presence – not even once. I chalked that up to a success.

PART IV: INTERNSHIP

Ch. 18:
A Glimpse Into the "Real World"

During my pediatrics/obstetrics rotation, I had the opportunity to apply for an internship that would span the majority of the upcoming summer. I was lucky enough to be accepted to the program and spent two full months working full-time hours in a medium-sized hospital in the midwest. Whereas in clinical I would usually not have more than six or seven hours per day on a unit with patients, for this internship, we were able to work three days per week, which were 12 hours each. While this was, indeed, a long shift, it represented what nurses in the "real world" manage to work. It also allowed all of us in the internship to be able to better understand the various stressors in the course of a shift that may occur and also helped us begin to prioritize our care, as we assumed care for a larger number of patients as the summer went on.

For this internship, we spent one month in one clinical area and then another month in some other area. While we were able to put in our preference for clinical areas, there was no guarantee we would be placed exactly where we wanted. We were also afforded several "special experience" days which allowed us to spend a day or two in a different area of the hospital. So that we had some guidance throughout our internship, we were each assigned a mentor to work with during our two rotations. In addition to our 36+ hours per week in the clinical setting, we spent five to six hours in a seminar-type class, where we discussed our experiences, completed simulations and worked on improving our approach to providing nursing care.

The first day of my summer internship was spent in a stuffy classroom, tucked away in the far corner of the hospital, getting to know the other students in the program. These students came from several states, and I knew a few students that attended my university. This first day was also the day that we were to find out what clinical assignements we would have. One by one, we were called up by the education coordinator to discuss our placement and schedule. It was nervewracking, not knowing our fate, and I couldn't help but feel a bit like Harry Potter being sent to the "sorting hat" to be told where I would end up.

As it turned out, the two clinical areas I was assigned included the cardiovascular unit and the house supervisor position. While the cardiovascular unit was pretty self-explanatory, the house supervisor had hospital-wide responsibilities. The house supervisor was in charge of staffing for the entire hospital for each shift, and he/she also had to respond to hospital emergencies, such as cardiac arrests, behavioral incidents and situations where patients' conditions were rapidly deteriorating. Both of these opportunities afforded me the chance to learn a lot about myself and working with patients.

Rapid Response

It was my fourth day with Mica, the house supervisor who I was assigned to. "Rapid response, room 1860, rapid response, room 1860, rapid response, room 1860," the intercom blasted. About that same time, Mica's pager began beeping obnoxiously. It read the same, "RAPID RESP--RM 1860."

More often than not, when a rapid response or cardiac arrest (not breathing, no pulse), was called, those responding did not know what they were responding to. A rapid response could be called for a variety of issues, from a patient having severe difficulty breathing to a person with a very low blood pressure. This morning was no different; we really had no idea what we were going to find when we got to the room.

We were moving down the hallways at a fast clip – not quite running but definitely moving faster than power walking – and I was about 3 strides behind Mica. "When we get there, you can just kind of melt into the wall, unless someone asks for something or you see something you can help with," he said.

We quickly entered room 1860, and there were already three nurses and a nursing technician there, along with one of the ER physicians who was busy giving orders. Apparently, the technician had found the older gentleman unresponsive and diaphoretic (sweaty) and called the rapid response. Upon further investigation, it was found that the patient only had a blood glucose level of less than 25. The machine that they used did not read any lower, and so there is no telling just how low the level actually was.

In reality, it didn't really matter – whether the glucose level was 2 or 20 mg/dL, the treatment for this patient would be the same – an "amp" (50 milliliters) of 50% dextrose to see if he could be aroused. This patient was getting 25 grams or about 100 Calories worth of glucose. If he responded fairly rapidly to that, his glucose level would be closely monitored, at least once every 15 minutes, until it got above 70 mg/dL. If he didn't respond fairly rapidly, an intravenous infusion of glucose would have been initiated in the IV line that had already been placed on the patient.

Luckily, this patient began to wake up, acting very groggy and disoriented, and asked what had happened. After it was clear that the patient was on the upswing and was having his sweat-soaked sheets changed, we headed back to the house supervisor office. Luckily, this patient did not require a rapid response any more during the shift.

Brief Encounters
"Here, you bag him while I get this cardiac monitor situated," stated the flight nurse, half out of breath. "See if you can get that CO2 down a little. He's at 46 now." She

had just climbed out of the helicopter, and the flight paramedic was busy getting the intravenous lines situated.

Mr. Simmons had been transferred by helicopter from a smaller hospital to the hospital I was doing my internship at because he required a higher level of care than could be provided at the smaller hospital. His medical issues were not very clear. Earlier in the afternoon, his sister had found him slumped over in his car seat. He did not appear to have had a heart attack, and the CT scan of the head did not show any sort of stroke. However, he was not breathing on his own, and he had to have a tube inserted into his airway.

I helped the nurse and paramedic get the patient situated on the gurney, and then we headed towards the intensive care unit. I bagged the patient the entire way there, and when we arrived, that was it. The respiratory therapist attached the endotracheal tube to the ventilator machine that was next to the patient's bed, and the ICU nurses began attending to the patient. For those short few minutes, I was delivering life-saving breaths of air to the patient, and then I went my separate way.

On the drive home from the hosital that night, I reflected on this interaction. Sometimes, nurses have days or even weeks in which to develop a rapport with patients. In this case, though, I had barely five minutes with the patient – and he was sedated. It was somewhat of a weird notion – that I could be in a critical role, keeping the patient alive, and then just dissapear from the patient's life.

Seizures

During my time in health care, I have occasionally felt somewhat helpless or that, regardless of what I did, I couldn't help the patient. That feeling was especially true the morning of my internship that I met Rakesh, a healthy-looking, athletic young man. The morning had been going well, and my preceptor, Dave, and I were making our rounds as normal.

At 30 years old, Rakesh had been married for three years to his lovely wife Cameron, and he had a one-year-old daughter, Kelsey. According to Cameron, he had been living a fairly normal life until he was twenty-nine. He had a seizure while out mowing the grass one day, but after being transported to the hospital, tests did not reveal any obvious cause for the seizure. Between that first seizure and the hospital admission when I took care of Rakesh, he had only two more seizures. This time, however, the situation seemed to be different.

Rakesh had been rushed to the hospital by paramedics after collapsing just before bed and going into a serious seizure, which lasted for 10 minutes in all. Cameron reported that his arm started twitching, and then his whole body seemed to come off of the ground. En route to the hospital, he was given a round of lorazepam, a benzodiazepine medication that is used to help stop seizures. Just as Rakesh was being wheeled into the emergency department doors, the seizures had ceased.

I assumed care for Rakesh the morning after this 10 minute seizure. When I walked in his room to introduce myself, I was greeted by his wife, Cameron, and both of his parents. It was only 7:00 AM, so having three visitors there already was a sign that the visitors cared about him (which is, unfortunately, not always the case). I said hello and performed my base head-to-toe assessment, which did not reveal any problems. Rakesh was in good spirits and seemed to be feeling just fine. As a precaution, the siderails of the bed had been padded, in case another seizure occurred.

After excusing myself and saying I would return in about an hour, I moved on to the next room, and Dave went with me. A few minutes later, Dave's work phone rang, and it was the unit clerk, telling her that Rakesh was having a seizure. Dave and I hurried to Rakesh's room. When I walked in, Rakesh's back was arched in a perfect upside down "u" shape. In fact, I remember thinking, "This man's back is going to break he's bent so much."

Rakesh had an as-needed dose of lorazepam ordered, so Dave quickly ran to the medication machine and withdrew the medication, drawing it up in a syringe and then administering it through his IV. At this point, Rakesh still had his back arched and his neck extended backward, and he was making whimpering noises, much like an animal that has been injured. His wife Cameron and his parents looked on in agony. Cameron had tears in her eyes and her hand placed on her mouth, shaking her head, while Rakesh's mother was at the head of the bed, trying to comfort him. About a minute after the lorazepam was given, he began to relax, and after about two more minutes, he came back around and was able to answer some questions.

"Did you notice anything different right before the seizure," I asked him.

"No. It just – it just happened," he replied. "I really wish that … that." And then his eyes began to roll back in his head, his arm started twitching, and he began to seize all over again.

Dave had dialed Rakesh's neurologist while I had been assessing him, and so he was actually on the phone during the seizure, explaining to the neurologist exactly what was happening. He instructed us to give Rakesh another dose of the lorazepam in hopes of stopping the seizure and advised that we could give another – but smaller – dose if it happened again. We gave the lorazepam, and it didn't seem to be touching the seizure, but after about two minutes, the seizure did let up again.

However, just like the first time, right after we started assessing Rakesh post-seizure, he went into another seizure. We gave the lorazepam as ordered, but again, it seemed that we were just waiting out the seizure and that the medication was doing no good. I felt useless. I was literally standing next to this patient's bed, watching him arch his back in what had to be terrible pain. I think his family felt equally as useless. Their soothing words were not helping him at all, and they had to watch as their loved one seized uncontrollably.

Dave called the neurologist again, and he made the decision to transfer Rakesh to the intensive care unit for closer monitoring and also to start him on a second mediation – phenytoin. We hurriedly wheeled him directly to the intensive care unit, just as he began what would be his fifth seizure of the morning, which lasted about three minutes.

After we got Rakesh to the intensive care unit and gave our report to the nurse there, we headed back to our unit. I found out later that afternoon that he was going to be transferred to a large metropolitan hospital for further evaluation and treatment, but to this day I have no idea what happened to him or if they discovered a specific cause for the seizures. That also makes it hard. So many times, when patients are transferred out of the unit that I am working on, I have no idea what happens to them. I would love to know if they pinpointed the cause of the seizures and were able to fix the problem, allowing Rakesh to live a seizure-free life. At the same time, I realize that it would have been likely a cause would never have been found and that he would be lucky if just the right cocktail of anticonvulsant medications would keep him in a stable, relatively seizure-free state.

One thing is for certain; I will never forget the sounds of agony that Rakesh made while having his seizures, and I will never forget the look on his family members' faces, especially when they looked at me as if to say, "Please help him. We beg you." There was nothing I could do but wait out the seizure and make sure he was still breathing and not choking.

PART V:
Medical-Surgical Nursing

Ch. 19:
The Semester of All Semesters

My summer internship taught me a lot, and I learned to organize myself more effectively, but the next semester of nursing school taught me many things as well. Indeed, it was the most difficult and taxing semester of them all. It was the semester of "med-surg."

From the time I entered nursing school, I heard about the infamous "med-surg" semester. Med-surg was short for "medical-surgical," and the focus of this clinical and lecture course was to teach us the essentials of caring for adult patients with medical problems, such as renal failure or pancreatitis, and surgical problems, such as an appendectomy or knee replacement. We would bounce between two hospitals for clinical and also do special experience days at other institutions and areas within the hospitals.

Several factors came together to make this semester so infamous. First, as if other semesters hadn't made sleep hard to get, this semester's demanding rigor led to few hours of sleep, which only made everything seem worse. Not only did we have a lot to get done, but we were frequently irritable and just wanted to crash on the bed, which was not really an option.

What caused this lack of sleep was clinical, which was probably one of the second major factors that made this semester infamous. From start to finish, we spent the better part of 24 hours devoted to a single patient and his or her care. A typical schedule for clinical, starting with the night before, looked like this:

- 4:00 – 6:00 PM: hospital to get patient information (All information, including admission history, diagnostic tests, plan of care, assessments, etc., had to be hand-written, which took forever, especially when patients had been there for several days – or weeks.)

- 6:30 – 7:00 PM: inhale supper
- 7:00 – 8:30 PM: type up patient's labs (I had a couple patients with 30+ tests, many of those repeated several times over a week) and diagnostic tests and the indication/significance of these studies
- 8:30 – 9:30 PM: type up patient's medications and drug information
- 9:30 – 11:00 PM: investigate the patient's diagnosis/problem and do relevant literature searches online and in textbooks
- 11:00 – midnight: develop a plan of care, with priority nursing diagnoses
- Midnight (hopefully): go to bed
- 4:45 AM: wake up
- 5:30 AM: at hospital reviewing chart and any changes that occurred overnight
- 6:00– 7:30 AM: pre-conference (We would be quizzed by our clinical instructor about our patients and our care plans. This was a stress-producing time, as the instructors grilled everyone to ensure they would be delivering safe, effective care.)
- 7:30 – 12:00 PM: clinical with patients
- 12:00 – 12:30 PM: post-conference

After we finished clinical in the early afternoon, we then had class from 2:00 PM until 4:00 PM, which many people fell asleep in because they were exhausted – physically and mentally. I then tutored from 4:00 PM to 6:00 PM and had a Student Senate meeting every Tuesday at 7:00 PM, which most certainly made for a long, long day.

Aside from clinical and sleep deprivation, the third component of the course, completing the "trifecta," if you will, was the sheer magnitude of lecture content for the classroom portion of the course. We had a ton of material to learn in just one semester, covering every body system and many different nursing concepts. Many students found themselves barely passing all semester long, which only added to the stress. They had made it to their next to last semester in nursing school, but would they be able to pass? Emotionally, this sent many students on a rollercoaster, again, not helped any by the lack of sleep that we were all faced with.

Even though med-surg had this "bad rap," I was interested to see if it would really be that bad. In the end, while I just wanted the semester to be over the entire time I was in the course, when I finished the semester, I knew I had accomplished something, and it felt good. I had overcome demanding lecture content and clinical, and I felt more prepared to be a "real" nurse.

Ch. 20:
Two Steps Forward,
Three Steps Backward

It was 4:00 PM, Monday – time to gather patient information for the first day of med-surg clinical. I had arrived at the hospital, not sure what I would find. After making my way to the tenth floor, I exited the elevator and walked towards the bustling nursing station, bracing myself for what patient would be written next to my name. Patient assignments were posted on a sheet in the break room, which was located immediately beside the nursing station. After entering the room, I turned to the right and looked up at the bulletin board, where the assignment sheet was tacked. There was the list, with our names typed and a patient name written right next to each of them. I scanned down the list. Dianne Winikie. She was to be my first med-surg patient.

As I exited the break room, I made my way towards the chart organizer to take a look at the patient's chart. "I wonder what she's here for," I thought to myself. "Will it be heart failure, pancreatitis, or something like pneumonia?" Leaning down, I selected the correct chart, which was chock-full of documents. The fact that the chart was overflowing with papers should have been my first clue that this patient had been there for quite some time and was also quite sick. I quickly flipped open the front cover of the chart. Glancing at the admission summary, my eyes found the admitting diagnosis section, which read "Admitted for 1) liver failure, 2) congestive heart failure, 3) COPD, 4) Alcoholism, 5) Colitis, 6) Chronic Renal Insufficiency."

"Holy cow," I said out loud – probably louder than I should have. I knew I was in for a long, long night.

"Well, I might as well start somewhere," I thought to myself. I logged into the computer, and by some miracle, the charting system let me in. Usually, logging into the hospital's charting system presented problems on the first clinical day, but not today. At least I had something going for me.

As this was my first medical surgical clinical, I was not very good at organizing my patient information collection process, so I did not really know what information I wanted to look at first, so I started at the labs. My eyes glanced through, literally, pages upon pages of lab results. "Oh for the love," I said, as Devon, one of the other nursing students walked up to see how I was doing. "This patient has had every damn test on planet earth done, and she has been here for almost two weeks. What is this madness?"

Devon just shook his head and said, "Dang. My patient only had a knee replacement, and he's only got a few labs and an x-ray."

Of course, in future weeks, I would have some of the "easier" patients like Devon's, but this week, I would be tested – physically and mentally.

Seven hours later, I was still working on clinical prep. It was 11:00 PM at this point, and I had finally finished up typing up all of the labs. I still had to type up the medication list (including the use for all of the medications, usual dosages, safety considerations, contraindications, nursing considerations, and so forth). Additionally, I had to type up a plan of care for the day, as well as summarize all, yes, all, of the conditions the patient was diagnosed with. By 3:00 AM, I had finished. All I had to do now was print out all of the documents I had created. Easy, right? No. It happened to be that night that my printer decided to malfunction. Instead of being able to print out the documents in my room, I had to walk across campus to one of the computer labs to print the material out. Still, it couldn't be easy. Both of the printers in the lab were down. At this point, so many explatives had exited my mouth that I don't think a case of soap could have washed my mouth out properly.

By some miracle, one of the other students that lived on my residence hall floor was awake and offered to let me print out the pages on his printer. To this day, I am forever grateful. That reduced my anxiety tremendously.

Now all of my material was prepared, and I could finally get sleep – an entire hour of sleep! Yes, at this point it was about 3:30 AM, and my alarm would be set for 4:30 AM so that I could get up, get ready, and be at the hospital by 5:30 AM.

Surprisingly, my brain actually woke me up when my alarm so annoyingly began to ring. I said a few explitives, cursed nursing school, sat up in bed, rubbed my eyes, and headed for the shower. About thirty minutes later, my truck was headed for the hospital.

We began pre-conference promptly at 6:00 AM in one of the conference rooms in the hospital, which seemed more like a death chamber than a place in which learning was to occur. Pre-conference was a sort of thrashing of each of us nursing students, one by one. Our professor, Dr. Lamb, sat at the end of the table, as each of us presented our patient to the rest of the group. After our first pre-conference, we were convinced her name was a façade. It was merely a cover for the wrath she would unleash upon us.

She frequently asked probing questions – so many questions that no matter how much we had prepared, we would not have all of the answers. "What complications will you be looking for in this patient?," she would ask. "Why might that be a complication? What kind of assessment will catch that complication? What do you have to make sure you do during that assessment that people forget to do most of the time? What will you do if you find that the person is having this complication? What lab tests might be ordered? Why would those lab tests be abnormal with that complication? What medication would you then give to help treat the complication? What is something major you have to remember when administering that medication? What will you be looking for after you give the medication? How will you know if the medication is important? Do you think your patient will need to be transferred to another unit for closer monitoring? Why don't you know that answer? You are the nurse, and you need to make sure you think about these things and are prepared." It wasn't abnormal for it to take half an hour to get through one patient.

At times, people cried. At times, people wanted to quit nursing. But in the end, even though Dr. Lamb demanded we "knew our stuff," we all had an extreme level of respect for her and her knowledge. There was a reason she was tough on us. After we left that clinical rotation with her, we felt more prepared to be nurses, not just average nurses but nurses that could critically think through scenarios in order to deliver excellent patient care. We would be proactive nurses – not reactive. Indeed, she made us realize that as nurses, we would have humans' lives in our hands, and we would be trusted to deliver the best care possible. She also cared about all of us and stood up for us. In a previous semester, she had even put a physician in his place after he accused a nursing student of making a mistake when it had actually been him who had made the mistake. Needless to say, she made it known that she was on our side. When we graduated, Dr. Lamb was smiling from ear to ear, happy to see us all walk across the stage.

But back to my patient. Ahh, yes. Ms. Winikie . . . My first med-surg patient and far and away the most complex case I dealt with during the semester. She was in her fifties, but she really looked much older – at least sixty five. Her hair was matted with a peculiar mix of gray and brown, and her abdomen was so distended from the liver failure, that she appeared to be pregnant.

Literally, it looked like she had placed a large watermelon in her abdominal cavity. Technically, this phenomenon is referred to as ascites (uh-site-ease). When a significant number of liver cells become damaged from chronic alcohol use, liver cirrhosis can develop, and when this occurs, pressures increase on the portal vein, a major blood vessel that carries blood to the liver to be filtered. When this pressure builds on the walls of the portal vein, fluid is pushed out of the vein into the abdominal cavity. To complicate matters, in patients with liver failure, blood protein levels tend to be low, and one function of protein in the blood is to help "pull" fluid into the vascular system, sort of like a sponge, and so with a lower protein level, it was even easier for fluid to stay out of the vascular system and remain in the abdominal cavity. Further, because of her heart failure, the heart muscle was not pumping effectively, and the kidneys were not functioning properly, resulting in even more fluid overload. Even worse, her COPD had been acting up and causing her to be short of breath all of her waking hours. To top it all off, she could not even think about eating any "real" food, as she was to have only clear liquids to "eat," given her colitis, an inflammation of the colon, many times treated by resting the bowel.

Perhaps what stood out most about Ms. Winikie were her eyes. I will never forget peering into her eyes and seeing despair and regret but also noticing how yellow they were. Indeed, I have seen many patients with scleral icterus – yellowing of the white part of the eye – but hers is still the worst I have ever seen. It seemed as if she were wearing colored contact lenses.

As I advanced into the room, I went through my typical introduction and then asked her how she was feeling. Though it wasn't actually a mistake to ask her this question, I sure felt like it was at the time.

"How in the hell do you think I'm feeling?" she asked accusingly. "I wouldn't be in this damn hospital, and I sure as hell would be eating, I mean drinking, more than this liquid piss. And here you come, asking me how I'm feeling, trying to make it all better. Who do you really think you are – just some nurse that is going to save the day, I'm sure. Well here's some free advice for you. Don't smoke. Don't drink. And don't take your body for granted."

Undoubtedly, I was taken aback by this short tirade, for lack of a better word. However, I noticed something in her voice, and I suppose I intuitively sensed some fear, sadness and worry in her. I have my excellent psychiatric-mental health rotation to thank for my ability to communicate with patients, and it most definitely helped in this situation.

"I'm sorry if I did not seem genuine in my question, but I really do want to help you feel better. I can't imagine what you are going through right now, but I want to do my best to make you better." I said this as sincerely as I possibly could. In the back of my mind, I knew that there was a lot I needed to talk with this patient about. Not only would I be tasked with trying to help her stop drinking and smoking, but I also needed to help her with her coping skills in general and also allow her to express her emotions of regret and sadness. I knew that I needed to establish good rapport with her first, so I simply said, "So tell me what is bothering you the most this morning. Maybe I can help you solve that problem or at least make it better."

To my surprise (I still wasn't sure if I was going to be met with stern resistance and a frown or would be allowed into her "world"), Ms. Winikie said that all she needed at that point was to breathe a little easier. "I just can't ever seem to catch my breath, and it leaves me feeling panicked. I don't like this big belly or this liquid diet or this diarrhea, but I don't like being short of breath more than all of that."

"I think we might be able to find some ways to help you a bit. For starters, have you ever tried pursing your lips like you are going to kiss someone?" I asked. "That helps you to exhale a bit more effectively; it gets more air out. Sometimes that can make a person feel better."

"Nah, I've heard something about it, but I've never really done that," she replied.

"Have you ever tried propping your arms in front of you and sitting like a tripod, in a way," I asked again.

"Nope. Never done that either," she responded.

"Can we try that now and just see what happens? All we can do is try," I suggested.

Sure enough, Ms. Winikie tried these two methods, and it did make a significant difference for her. I had seen it help a little in the past but never as much as it seemed to with Ms. Winikie. I'm not sure if part of it was in her head – that she was psychologically convinced she was short of breath – but pursed lipped breathing and the tripod position sure helped her.

"Wow," she said, after about a minute. "I think I'm going in the right direction with this. I don't feel like I'm gasping."

In addition to these two techniques, when it was time for her morning medications, she was to take an inhaler. "Before you take this inhaler," I said, "I would love for you to show me how you normally do your inhaler. Can you walk me through the process? I know it might seem like a funny question, but inhalers these days are so confusing at times, and I want to make sure you're getting the full benefit of it."

"Well I guess," she responded, sounding somewhat perplexed. "Well, while I'm breathing, I just squeeze the inhaler, like this." That was her only step in administering the inhaler.

Taking an inhaler properly actually involves several important steps. First, the inhaler should be shaken, in order to ensure the contents are mixed and available when the canister is squeezed. Second, it's important to exhale as much as possible (which is admittedly difficult for a patient with COPD) prior to squeezing the inhaler so that when inhaling, the lungs are able to pull more of the medication in. Additionally, the inhaler should actually be held about an inch from the mouth – not placed inside the mouth. Finally, once the inhaler is squeezed and the medication is in the lungs, it is important for the patient to hold his or her breath for 10 seconds, or as long as possible if a patient isn't able to make it to 10 seconds.

It was fairly obvious to me that Ms. Winikie missed all of these important steps, and I discussed the proper method of using an inhaler with her. I also explained why each step was important, so that she could see what I was saying was not a bunch of unimportant excess. I then had her demonstate for me the proper way to use an inhaler, which she got right for the most part, although she did forget to hold her breath for 10 seconds.

"I think if you keep working on that, you will probably find that the inhaler works a bit better for you," I commented.

"Well, I sure hope so," she responded.

Indeed, when I came back on Thursday, she reported that she felt like the inhalers had been working, though by that point, another complication had arisen.

After this respiratory education, I needed to complete a head-to-toe assessment on Ms. Winikie which went smoothly. She was the "perfect patient" as I listened to her heart, lung and bowels with my stethoscope, looked at her pupils with my pen light, and tapped on her abdomen, seeing if I could produce a "fluid wave" from the ascites in her belly.

After the assessment, I decided to take a small risk and try to delve a little more into what she was feeling emotionally and psychologically. "So how has this hospitalization affected you?" I asked. "Since I've never been in your shoes, I'd like to try to get a better understanding of what you are going through."

"Well. We are all going to die some day, I guess," she replied.

"Die?" I thought to myself. I didn't say anything about death.

"But I don't want it to be now. I don't want it to be ten years from now," she continued. "I just wish I wouldn't have been stupid. I've been so selfish and had so much fun all of these years, and I can't take it back now."

"Can't take it back now?" I queried.

"Yeah. There's no way I can undo what I've done – all the smoking, drinking, partying," she replied.

"Well there are certainly ways to help prevent worsening and get you back to a level where you can at least have a better quality of life than what you're having now," I responded. "Maybe in a bit we can talk about those," I suggested, which she seemed agreeable to. (Later that day, we had a lengthy discussion about those very strategies. She had not considered that stopping smoking and drinking could have any positive benefit. She had always been told her conditions were chronic and permanent, and so she assumed quitting would have no positive benefit at all, which wasn't correct.)

"So it sounds like at this point you are afraid of the possibility of death," I said.

"Yea. And it's not really dying as much as it is what would happen if I died," she responded.

"Mmmhmm," I replied. "Can you tell me more about what you mean by that?"

"Well I have six children," she responded. "And they're still growing up. I still have so much I want them to know, and I want to be a better example for them. I feel like I have let them down."

"I wonder if there is something you could do now that might help show them how to live life well," I replied. "What would you like them to see in you right now?" I asked. "What are things that you have control over right now that you could change in your life?"

We then spent the next 30 minutes discussing coping strategies and ways to reflect positivity. We also talked about positive things in her life – her strengths and resources. As it turned out, she was very religious, and she found a lot of solace considering her religion and talking with the pastoral care personnel at the hospital. She also had a sister who loved her dearly and was a shining spot in her life. Finally, we talked about her children and how she could be a good role model for them from the point of hospitalization forward.

After the lengthy discussion, we agreed that she should probably get a bit of rest, as she was to have physical and occupational therapy a little bit later in the day. I then went off to chart my assessment findings and continue brainstorming ways to help her.

By the end of the shift, I felt like I had made a significant impact on Ms. Winikie's life, and I was excited to come back Thursday to continue working with her. She would be in the hospital several more days, as she was scheduled for a paracentesis, a draining of the fluid in her abdomen, the next day, and she also needed additional treatment for her heart failure.

When I came back Thursday, my plan of care for that day was blown out of the water, as her condition had changed – for the worse.

I arrived Thursday at about 5:40 AM, and Dr. Lamb waved me over to where she was sitting. "Hey, make sure you take a peak at your patient's chart from after you were here getting updates on her last evening – especially the labs. It looks like they are probably going to send her over to the ICU."

"Oh, great," I thought to myself. "What happened now?"

After a brief review of the chart, I found out that at about 4:00 AM, Ms. Winikie began having severe chest pain, followed by an increased need for oxygen. After running several lab tests and doing a CT of the chest, it was found that she had suffered from a pulmonary embolism, where a blood clot lodged in one of the blood vessel branches in the lungs, making proper blood flow through the lungs difficult. While she was still breathing, and her oxygen levels were doing okay, she needed to be watched very closely, as her respiratory status could worsen fairly easily. As Dr. Lamb had suggested, about that time the hospitalist physician came around and told the nurse that he was going to move Ms. Winikie to the ICU.

At that point, I went to her room to say that I was thinking about her and also wished her luck. "Remember what we talked about Tuesday," I said sincerely.

Even in her shortness of breath from the pulmonary embolism, she still managed a half smile and simply said, "Thanks."

I'm not sure what ended up happening with Ms. Winikie. I never had the opportunity to care for her again, and I couldn't look through files later, as this would be a violation of patient privacy, since I was no longer taking care of her; it would have just been out of pure curiosity which was not a valid reason to obtain additional patient information.

To this day, I still think about that one word – "Thanks." It means a lot to this day. It's not that I need to be thanked every single time I take care of a patient; no, this is my job, after all. However, when a patient thanks me, it is a signal that I made a difference for him or her, and that is what I valued in nursing school and what I still value to this day – simply (or not so simply) making a difference, whether it is a small difference or large difference.

Ch. 21:
Being Present . . .

Betty Wortzler was dying, and she knew it. At 62 years old, she had just become a grandmother and wanted to do anything she could to enjoy some time with her new arrival. For almost three decades, she lived with the knowledge that she suffered from multiple sclerosis, commonly called MS.

Put simply, MS makes the body's nervous system much less effective at transmitting any signals. On the outside of nerves is a coating, much like the coating on electricity lines. This coating helps nerve signals be transmitted efficiently, as they are more or less "contained" in this wrapping, so the signal only has one direction in which to go, and it can't diffuse widely. In MS, however, this coating begins to be broken down, making it difficult for signals to be quickly and efficiently disseminated along the nerve route. Different types of MS exist, and some persons experience more severe symptoms than others, however. Unfortunately for Ms. Wortzler, though, she had a particularly insidious form. She had lost a significant amount of voluntary muscle control and had trouble even feeding herself, as her arms and hands would shake too much. But the MS wasn't what was going to kill her; it was her terrible heart function.

About a month and a half prior to this hospitalization, Ms. Wortzler had suffered a massive heart attack, referred to as a ST-segment elevation myocardial infarction. She had been feeling extremely tired for a couple weeks prior to this event, but she just chalked it up to being run down from her MS. Unfortunately, this fatigue was a warning sign of an impending cardiac event. The heart attack left her with her heart muscle functioning at a very low level, making if quite difficult for her body's pump (the heart) to keep up with the amount of fluid flowing through the vascular system. In turn, blood was backing up into the lung's blood vessels, causing pulmonary (lung) congestion, and also causing a significant amount of fluid to accumulate in the air "sacs" in the lung, called pulmonary edema. This, of course, was making it extrememly difficult for her to breathe properly.

Physicians had tried many things to help her heart and reduce the amount of fluid in her body, but it seemed it would only be a matter of time before she would succumb to her illness. Today, my goal would be to keep her alive a little longer – until her son and new granddaughter could make it to see her from California. They were to arrive late that evening.

Starting my day, I knew it was going to be an emotionally difficult one. In prioritizing my care for the day I was balancing two pieces. I needed to ensure that she could have as comfortable a death as she could have mentally, but to do that, I also had to focus on managing her symptoms and keeping her alive physically. Thus, not only would I focus significantly on her psychosocial well-being, but I also had to ensure I was carrying out orders and providing physical nursing care quite effectively.

After pre-conference, I dropped off a few unnecessary items in the break room and took a deep breath. While I knew it was my duty to take care of this patient, I wasn't particularly enthusiastic about it, because I knew how short of a time it seemed she had left to live. What would I say? How would I act? Of course, I had rehearsed scenarios in my head the night before and that morning, but I couldn't control what Ms. Wortzler would say. What if she sobbed uncontrollably? What if she refused to interact with me?

Looking back, I was lucky to have had a fantastic psychiatric-mental health course during nursing school, and I think that this course helped prepare me for the communication skills I would need in interacting with Ms. Wortzler. Additionally, my sophomore year of college, I had read a book called *Final Gifts: Understanding the Special Awareness, Needs, and Communications of the Dying*, written by Maggie Callanan and Patricia Kelley, both nurses who worked in hospice care. This book had given me more perspective on working with hospice patients and their families. (Interestingly, this book was given to me by a professor I had for several classes during college, Kay White, who is a licensed clinical social worker who spent many years in the hospital, working right alongside patients. She must have known it would come in handy for me, and it did.)

At any rate, I knew it was time.

I walked into her room and introduced myself. She graciously welcomed me and said, "Well how did you end up with me as a patient – such a pain in the butt?"

"You're my only focus today, and you can be as big a pain in the butt as you want. I'm yours." She smiled and nodded.

I then examined her, gave her her morning medications and then proceeded to spend nearly four hours just sitting in her room next to her. She was very weak and barely had any energy to talk, so I offered to just sit with her and be present as she waited for her family to arrive. We did make some small talk, but the essential message she kept giving me was "please just stay here." It amazed me how much just being present with someone meant. She knew very little about me, other than the fact that I was a nursing student, but she valued my presence. Not being alone meant the world to her.

That day, I didn't do anything invasive (like starting an IV or inserting a Foley catheter or nasogastric tube). I did not give any powerful IV medications, and I did not have to change multiple dressings. All I did was sit in a chair next to a patient's bed, and this had made a difference. Sometimes, it really is the small things, like just being present, that make the biggest difference.

Ch. 22:
On a Happy Note . . .

From the stories I've already told in this portion of the book, it probably seems like my medical-surgical rotation was full of sad accounts of deathly ill patients who had little positive in their lives. However, this rotation also introduced me to several very interesting characters.

Ms. Dubose

Martha Agnes Dubose. Ah, yes. This centenarian, clocking in at 104 years young, was a spitfire, no doubt about it. She had broken her arm in four distinct places due to a crash she incurred while riding an adult tricycle. It wasn't her fault, though, she had insisted; it was the "nimrod who left a bunch of sticks on the sidewalk." Apparently, she had been riding her three-wheeled bike and hit a patch of brush on the sidewalk, causing her bike to get caught in a rut between the sidewalk and grass. She had been jolted off to the side of the bike, lost her balance, and fell to the ground.

After a quick surgery, which was quite risky at her age, I was taking care of her on a surgical floor. I knew who was in charge the second I walked in the room, and I had no time to even introduce myself.

"Oh, hello, young man," she quipped as I walked through the door. "I am Ms. Martha A. Dubose, and it's nice to meet you. I see you are a nursing student, according to your uniform. We will get along famously this morning, as long as you help me accomplish two tasks. First, I would like some fresh towels, a comb and some new foam soap to help me freshen up. Second, if you could find out what channel the horse racing is on, that would be marvelous."

I didn't know quite what to think. Generally, as a student nurse, I was used to guiding the conversation, at least initially. This was clearly not the case with Ms. Dubose. No, she knew what she wanted, and she let me know about it.

She was also a tough 104-year-old. During the whole affair, she had taken perhaps two or three pain pills at most. She insisted that she felt fine and that she had experienced much more severe pain in her life. It astounded me at the time. I was used to people with this sort of fracture and surgery asking for copious pain medications, including intravenous medications. Not for Ms. Dubose, however; she was in control.

We did get along "famously" that day, as she had suggested. In fact, she provided three what she called, "secrets to a long life"
1. Good family
2. Handsome husband
3. Nice kids.

"It just that simple," she suggested. "People get all googly-eyed about things in the world today. Why? There's no point in it. Just enjoy the positive in life."

Sometimes, no, many times, patients provide nurses and nursing students with more to think about than just medical issues and medications, and Ms. Dubose was surely one of them. During a busy semester, with a lot going on in my academic and personal life, her words came at an opportune time, and I appreciated them greatly.

"Billy"

Billy Anderson was set in his ways and knew what worked – at least he thought he did. I only worked with Mr. Anderson for a short time, as I was leading a team of nursing students, and one of my fellow students, Stephanie, was his primary student nurse.

"You have to go see this guy," Stephanie insisted. "Just go talk to him, and you'll understand," she continued, with a smile from ear to ear.

After I had checked in with the other members of the student nurse team, I headed to "Billy's" room. He actually insisted on being called Billy. "If you're going to call me Mr. Anderson, you might as well leave. I'm Billy – always have been and always will be. Mr. Anderson is my father."

Billy was 76.

After a brief introduction, I asked him how he was feeling.

"Well, you see," he started in, "I'm feeling great now. Do you know why I'm feeling great now?" Billy questioned.

"Not exactly," I responded. "Tell me about it."

He shook a salt packet he had somehow coaxed out of one of the food service personnel that delivered his breakfast tray.

"What in the world…?" I thought to myself.

"I figured out how to take care of all this pain I've been having, and you wouldn't believe it. These pharmaceutical companies, they just want to make a bunch of money, ya' know. They don't really want to help us. They are out to make a buck. Never trust those guys. Believe me. But, anyway, my wife, she called me from home because I couldn't remember what kind of medicine I had been taking off and on at home to help my pain, and the nurses last night were asking me what it was, but of course I couldn't remember because my brain gets all jumbled like it's full of a bunch of mud, but yeah, anyway, my wife, ya' know what she said? She said it was naproxen sodium," he said in an exasperated tone.

Naproxen sodium is commonly called Aleve or Naprosyn, and it is a common over-the-counter pain reliever. Billy went on, though, to explain why he was so upset with pharmaceutical companies.

"Sodium. Can you believe that? All these years I've been buying salt. Salt for heaven's sake. What is this world coming to?"

Billy thought that the "sodium" portion of naproxen sodium meant that he was taking salt tablets, as sodium and salt meant the same thing to him. In fact, the active ingredient is the naproxen part of the medication, and sodium is just a component of the chemical structure. He had concluded that taking a packet of salt would be the same as taking a naproxen sodium tablet.

"And guess what," he said, challenging me.

"What?" I replied with a smile.

"It works. I got those suckers good. No more pain for me."

I then spent twenty minutes trying to explain the pharmacology of naproxen sodium and the difference between the sodium in naproxen and the sodium portion of table salt, but I made no progress. He was convinced he had uncovered one of the biggest plots of the century.

I politely excused myself and went to find Stephanie, who had been charting her assessment and writing a short progress note on Billy.

"You'll never believe the conversation I just had," I said in a disbelieving tone.

"Oh, great," she responded. "I can only imagine. He sure is an interesting man."

I explained the situation to Stephanie, and she decided to focus her care plan for the day on educating Billy.

"That might be the most difficult care plan of the century," I noted, smirking jokingly with her.

She just shook her head and said, "I better get started."

Stephanie never did convince Billy. Our only recourse was to let the RN taking care of Billy know about the situation. She decided to put a referral in for a pharmacist to come talk to him, but I doubt that worked either. He was probably convinced that the pharmacist was in cahoots with the pharmaceutical companies.

While this story is somewhat entertaining, it also illustrates an important issue in society – health literacy. Many patients have their own beliefs about health care, and many have significant trouble interpreting medical information. It is essential for health care personnel to evaluate patients' understanding of medical and health-promotion topics in order to ensure that they receive the best care possible and that they truly understand how to care for themselves.

Ch. 23:
Stress and Anxiety, Part 2

Med-surg reminded me that I *had* to take time for myself to relax and also to express my emotions.

One of the most unique aspects about nursing school was that we were not only having to deal with the emotion that goes along with college and transitioning to a new phase in our lives, but we also were experiencing the very real emotions of our patients and their familes. We saw patients die; we saw patients cry; we saw families hug their loved one, not knowing if they would see them alive again; we worked with patients that had attempted suicide multiple times; and we talked with homeless persons whose only fault in life was being victimized and left on the street as a child. Indeed, the emotion that we had to process and then express ourselves was complex.

For me, relaxation took several forms, most notably *doing absolutely nothing* other than sitting on the couch and watching TV. I didn't even need anyone else to be present. In fact, a lot of the time, I preferred to be alone.

Many weekends, I traveled back to my hometown to spend time relaxing. This included "hanging out" with my grandparents and other family members. I also would sometimes meet up with old friends from high school or just "chill" on the couch. Getting off campus and back to my hometown represented a sort of "escape" for me. While I absolutely loved spending time at Millikin, I also needed some time away, which these weekend vacations allowed for. When I was home, I did not feel the need to impress anyone; I didn't have to live with any roommates; it wasn't necessary for me to engage in social groups (if I just felt like being alone); and I could see my family and catch up with them. I did receive quite a lot of flack for this decision to come home on the weekends, but to this day, I realize that it is what I needed at the time.

I also found that journaling helped me tremendously. As readers can probably tell from the pages of this book, being a nursing students is a very emotional experience. It is not always – in fact, rarely is it – fun. It's tough, and it takes a toll on a person's emotions. I needed a way to express this emotion, and journaling allowed me to express these feelings. When I didn't have the time to hand-write my entries, I would create journaling videos that allowed me to process emotions verbally but not have to spend the extra time commiting those words to paper.

Aside from journaling and having my "sanity" time on the weekends, I also vented to my fellow nursing students. We all vented, in fact. Most of us found that our other friends and family members did not entirely understand what we were going through. Sometimes we would meet after clinical and talk about our day, while other times, we would all meet for a group meal and movie night – spending most of this time talking about our lives. These were some of the most memorable, rewarding and cathartic moments of nursing school.

Ch. 24:
The Intensive Care Unit

One special experience that I looked forward to all semester during med-surg was my rotation in the intensive care unit. I had not been able to spend any time around intensive care units in the past, so this was to be a new experience for me, and I was quite interested in learning about ventilators (breathing machines) and proper management of patients on one of these machines. As it turned out, I would learn about ventilator managment with the very first patient I took care of in the unit.

The intensive care unit (ICU) was somewhat of a different world. Instead of several lengthy hallways, with patient rooms scattered about, the entensive care unit was more like a block of rooms in a rectangle. The nurses station was located in the middle of this block, so that help was never more than a few steps away. Nurses could view several screens scattered around the desks with each patient's heart monitor and latest vital signs displayed. A fairly consistent "bing, bing, bing," and the occasional high pitched "ding, ding, ding" could be heard from these machines, alerting nurses to potential problems with their patients. Most of the time, it was more or less a "false alarm," but each time the alarm went off, it definitely made me look at the monitor, even though it never once tunred out to be anything serious during my time in the ICU.

In addition, nursing in the ICU was slightly different. The nurses had one or two patients usually and ocassionally three, if one of the patients was soon going to be transferred to a different floor and was more stable. While the challenge on some general nursing units is balancing out the care of seven, eight or more patients at once, in the ICU, the challenge is that each patient (generally) has to have frequent assessments, medications and special nursing care, such as suctioning, ventilator management, and central line dressing changes/care (not that this does not occur in other units, but it is particularly prevalent in the ICU).

After arriving about 20 minutes early, at 5:40 AM, I was ready to get the day going, but I had to wait for my ICU preceptor for the day, Matt, to arrive. After ten minutes of waiting, I saw a rather portly, middle-aged man walk into the main doors of the unit. As he came closer, I could see that his name tag said Matthew, and after the unit clerk confirmed that he was indeed my preceptor, I walked up and introduced myself.

"Hi," I said. "My name is John, and I'm a nursing student from Millikin. I'm supposed to work with you today."

"Pleased to meet, ya, young man," Matt replied. He had a touch of southern accent to his voice, and it sounded like he might have grown up somewhere outside of Central Illinois. "How are you this fine morning?," he asked.

"I'm doing just fine. I'm ready to see some new things," I replied. "How are you?"

"Oh, I'm doing fair to middlin', I suppose. I can't complain when I've got it so much better than any one of these patients in these parts [the ICU]," he retorted. "Well, shall we see our patients for the day?" he asked, more or less indicating that is what we were going to do.

For the ICU experience, I was to be more or less a shadow – a shadow that was supposed to ask as many questions as possible, soak in nursing practice in the ICU and perform nursing interventions that I had been "checked off" on previously. While we had a nursing instructor present on another unit in the hospital, we were essentially on our own, only working with the preceptor.

On this day, we would have two patients. First, we met Della Worthington, an older lady that had been found unconscious and unresponsive at her home, though she was breathing. On the way to the hospital, she went into respiratory arrest and needed to have oxygen pumped into her lungs via a tube placed in her airway. A chest x-ray, bloodwork, and other lab tests showed that the patient had severe pneumonia, and she was known to have severe COPD, making the pneumonia more dangerous, given that COPD makes it much more difficult to expel mucous secretions from the lungs.

Our goal for the day would be to try to see if we could get the patient off of the ventilator, or breathing machine, that she was on. We would be performing what is known as a "weaning trial," a way to test the patient's readiness for coming off of the ventilator. After performing other assessments and ensuring that the family understood what was happening, we began the weaning trial, which involved reducing the amount of sedative the patient was receiving and also adjusting the ventilator settings, eventually allowing the patient to breathe on her own accord, as much as possible.

With this patient, it was interesting to see her go from sedated to conscious during the weaning trial, where I was, in a sense, able to get to know her, communicating via a note pad. She couldn't communicate with me verbally, given she had a breathing tube still present in her throat. During the weaning trial, I spent a lot of my time in Ms. Worthington's room, talking to her and trying to keep her as calm as possible, as she was very anxious about being intubated. The patient's lung sounds left a lot to be desired; she had some wheezing and crackles throughout the lung fields, and we were focusing on getting her sitting up, providing suction, and providing good oral care.

Unfortunately, because COPD makes exhaling air more problematic, carbon dioxide (CO_2) was building up in the patient's lungs and not being expelled during normal expiration. We checked Ms. Worthington's blood to see what her CO_2 and oxygen levels were, among other things, and, regrettably, we found that she indeed was building too much

CO2, even though her oxygen level was okay. Even given that sufficient oxygen was reaching her lungs, the excess CO2 that was also present caused the pH level in her blood to become more acidic, which is a dangerous situation. For this reason, she was immediately put back on the ventilator.

Our second patient, Mr. Sunland, was admitted after having been on another unit for gastroenteritis, an inflammation in the digestive system. The nurses on that unit found him having significant breathing problems, and intubation was performed. This intubation took an extended amount of time, however, because the patient was morbidly obese and had significant tracheal edema, swelling of the tube in the neck that goes to the lungs. Having been in the ICU for three days already, Mr. Sunland was now breathing fairly well with only oxygen delivered to his nose. He no longer needed the tube in his airway.

However, because of the extra time it took to get life-saving oxygen to the patient initially, there was concern that the patient could have experienced some degree of anoxic encephalopathy, which is a fancy way for saying part of the brain could have been negatively impacted by a lack of oxygen, resulting in deficits in normal function. Indeed, Mr. Sunland required help in all activities of daily living, meaning that we had to help him do basically everything a "healthy" person would do in a day – bathing, dressing, eating, and so forth. He was also somewhat confused, and at one point, he began swinging at us as we were trying to provide him with a bath.

"Let's give him a minute to relax," Matt suggested. "At this point, it is not cruicial we give him a bath because he did get one yesterday evening, and he may just want to be left alone for a little while. We can try again later."

This sounded like a plan to me. Matt was correct. We returned to Mr. Sunland's room about two hours later, and he was more than happy to receive a bath. In fact, he even smiled when we walked in the room with bathing supplies.

My first day in the ICU was actually fairly uneventful, though I learned a lot talking to Matt and exploring the various protocols used in the unit. I also was looking forward to coming back on Thursday – hoping I would have the same patients.

When I returned Thursday, Matt was the charge nurse for the ICU, so he only had one patient, but, luckily, I was back with Ms. Worthington. What a joy it was to work with her on Thursday. Luckily, she was extubated on Wednesday with no complications, and when I first visited her in the morning on Thursday, she had just been taken off of a biphasic positive airway pressure (bi-pap) machine, basically a mask that fits on the face and helps to manipulate pressure in the airway to allow for proper ventilation of the lungs. She was on oxygen running in her nose at this point, and after a couple hours, we drew blood to see how much CO_2 she was retaining. Today, her lab values were much better.

As compared with just two days prior, this patient was smiling and joking around with hand gestures, even though she was not talking too much. Her throat was still quite sore from the tube that was used during intubation. The paramedic had used a larger than normal size ET tube when he/she intubated the patient in the ambulance, so the RN said this could play a role in the sore throat as well. She was so very appreciative of the care that was being provided, and it was truly inspiring to see this patient from being on a ventilator to being transferred out of the ICU. Because this patient had made so much progress and only needed to be on oxygen delivered through the nose, it was decided that she was well enough to go to a step-down medical floor. Towards the end of the clinical day, the tech and I transferred her to this medical floor, and I was able to wish her a speedy recovery.

Mr. Sunland, whom I worked with on Tuesday, was transferred to a general medical floor on Wednesday, but I'm not sure what became of him after that point. I certainly hope that he made improvements, but brain injuries are insidious animals, and it's many times difficult to predict exactly how well a patient will do.

After my special experience days in the ICU, I had a much better understanding of what it was like to work in such a setting, but I had mixed feelings. While it was indeed rewarding to see patients get better, there were also many patients who were quite ill – many of whom did not have good outcomes.

PART VI: COMMUNITY HEALTH NURSING

Ch. 25: "Call 911 . . ."

Many of the lessons I learned while in community health, I never would have expected, especially the lessons I learned on a cold, February day.

I walked in the door, knowing that the patient had fallen but not knowing much else. While I was in a hurry, I wasn't emergently concerned. My adrenaline hadn't really kicked in too much, since it was just after 6:00 AM.

I had gone through situations in my head: If he is having significant pain, or if he had hit his head, we would call 911 and try to get any fractures stabilized. On the other hand, if it was more of a controlled fall, and he was just having trouble getting up, I'd opt to try to get him up on my own first and then go from there on my assessment. I knew he was not on a blood thinner like warfarin, so I wasn't terribly concerned about internal bleeding, either.

I walked in, and his wife was standing in the living room, as she knew I was coming. "Hi, John. Sorry to get you up early. He's in the bathroom," she said.

I sat my medical bag on the small couch off to the right and made my way the few steps down the short hallway to the left. As I glided my way down the hallway, an odd vibe came over me. I'm not really sure how to describe it, but it was there – a sort of ethereal feeling of unrest.

As I walked into the bathroom, I found the patient lying on his left side, with his head lying limp, slightly angled towards the ground. He had a white undershirt on, along with his underwear, but nothing else. He wasn't moving. His legs had a mottled, cobblestone-like appearance.

I didn't like what I saw, and I felt my adrenaline start to rev up. I called out his name two or three times, but there was no response, so I instructed my partner to call 911 and tell them that we had an 86-year-old male that was unresponsive.

From this point forward, I went on autopilot. There is no other way to describe it.

I turned the patient to his back and did a hard sternal rub on the center of his chest, trying to elicit some sort of response, but there was none. I immediately checked for a pulse at the patient's carotid artery, in the valley about halfway between the side of the neck and the trachea, which was absent. It was obvious at this point that he wasn't breathing either, as his chest was not rising, and I could hear no respirations.

I yelled to my partner to "tell them he is not breathing and has no pulse – CPR in progress." I knew I had a bag-valve mask in my medical bag (one of the tools that are commonly seen in television shows and movies when medical personnel are "bagging" a patient – squeezing a football-looking bag that is delivering air to the patient), and I knew that the patient's wife was on oxygen at night and had a portable oxygen tank.

I ran to grab the portable tank and also my bag-valve mask and very quickly hooked up the bag to the oxygen. This took maybe 20 seconds, as I was in turbo mode. By that time, my partner had gotten off the phone with 911 and was back at the bathroom. "Here, you do airway and bag," I said, as I started compressions.

"One, two, three . . ." I counted rapidly as I compressed the patient's chest. I could feel a crack here and there – likely ribs cracking under the pressure of my compressions. To be quite honest, in retrospect, the feeling of ribs cracking was not nearly as bad as I had anticipated. People had told me that I would feel this but made it seem so much worse than it really was.

We got into a rhythm, doing compressions and delivering blasts of oxygenated air to the patient, and I began to think about what else we needed to do. I realized he still had his shirt on, so I yelled for a pair of scissors, which the patient's wife brought. During a rescue breath, I cut off the patient's shirt and then began compressions again.

It seemed like it took forever and a day, but paramedics soon arrived. Actually, it only took them 4 or 5 minutes from the time 911 was dialed until they pulled up. Nonetheless, I was sweating and getting winded from doing compressions for just this relatively short time.

I began to give the paramedics a report of what had happened, including the patient's history and what we had done. They quickly dragged him to the living room and dropped him onto the spine board. From that point on, the paramedics ran the code. On the cardiac monitor, he was in asystole, meaning that there was essentially no electrical activity in the heart. The paramedics started giving epinephrine and atropine trying to get some electrical activity in the heart and then transported the patient to the local hospital.

We met them at the hospital. I knew that things didn't look good, and I was right. About fifteen minutes after arriving at the hospital, my grandpa was pronounced dead.

It was such a surreal moment, and to this day, I am astounded by what transpired that morning. The "partner" that I had was actually my mom, who was CPR certified in her role as a school teacher. She knew what to do, just like I did. The patient's wife, of course, was my grandma.

Never did I think the first person I would perform CPR on would be my grandpa. However, I learned so very much from this experience.

I learned that, in crisis situations, I can stay focused and push my emotions aside to do what needs to be done when it needs to be done and worry about the emotion later. While this may sound somewhat unaffected or indifferent, in fact, it is necessary. Too much emotion on the part of rescuers in life and death situations is not good for the patient; they need to be resuscitated, period. After the fact, my friends and family asked me how I could do what I did.

"I just did," I would say. "There is no real way to describe how it happened. I just went into 'go' mode and did what I had to do."

Looking back, it is my training and scenario simulations that really got me through. I had been CPR certified for almost seven years and had renewed my certification several times. Further, I had practiced cardiac arrest simulations during school. In my mind, I had gone through what I would do in different situations, and an in-home cardiac arrest was one of these scenarios. I was ready, plain and simple.

While it was a very unfortunate day, and one that I recalled before I went to bed for almost two months after and dreamt about on and off for over a year, perhaps the final gift that my grandpa gave me was knowing that I could do what was necessary in these grave situations. It also provided me with valuable reminders. Truthfully, I think that we did almost everything right. The only minor aspect of that morning that I would have changed would have been to pull my grandpa into the living room immediately, instead of staying in the bathroom. That would have given us more room to work, not that this made a huge difference. I also probably should have started compressions immediately, not deviating to grab the oxygen tank and mask, though it would have been difficult for anyone else to have located the bag-valve mask in my medical bag. Fast (at least 100 per minute), hard compressions are by far and away the most important component of CPR in the community setting.

One reason that I told this story at first, as if the patient was someone I was assigned through nursing school, was because I wanted to reveal one way that I was able to get through the situation. I broke everything down into very basic parts: I had a patient (not my grandfather) who had a medical emergency that needed to be addressed. I was a trained nursing student (not a grandson) who could do something. It's as simple as that.

At the same time, I hope that telling the story the way I did put into perspective what families go through. The situation showed me how "real" health care is and how we can sometimes forget how critical it is to help comfort families in their times of grief and sorrow. As I paced around the emergency department and down the main hallway of the hospital, trying to find some sort of intangible solace, I looked around at all of the people going to and coming from their physician appointments. I saw nurses and doctors walking around, taking care of patients and attending to the needs of others. Their day was only minorly impacted by the death of my grandpa. Their day still went on as "normal." The world itself continued to spin. But mine had been turned upside down. My life had changed forever.

While we (as health care personnel) can sometimes break things down into their basic parts – a lifeless human body devoid of emotion and personality – in order to make it through situations, we have to acknowledge the emotion involved. When we arrived at the hospital that morning, so many personnel hugged me and gave me words of encouragement; to this day I am immensely grateful. I knew many of the staff in the emergency department, and one of the nurses, Lisa, was talking to me outside of the resuscitation room. The doctor had just stuck his head out and essentially told me that things looked very bad, and I was getting ready to go tell my family the news. "Would you like me to go with you, John?" she asked?

At the time, I said, "No. I'll be okay." Even though I really wanted her to go with me.

Somehow, she just knew I needed the support. I walked away from the resuscitation room towards the family waiting room, and she trailed behind. When we got to the room, she was there for moral support and even helped explain some of what was going on. She talked to me a little longer and patted me on the shoulder, telling me I would be okay – that I was smart, driven and that I would make a difference in the world and make my grandpa proud. That morning, I realized just how important compassion in health care can be.

Ch. 26:
"Why would you want to do *that*?"

I was sitting in a classroom before class had begun. There were about ten other students in the room carrying on conversations and sharing the latest gossip. As it so happened, the topic for the day was older adults, aging, and community resources, and everyone had printed out the PowerPoint presentation slides for that day.

Many times when I have told people I enjoy working with geriatric patients, I have gotten the "disgusting" face . . . the squinted eyes, scrunched up nose, and semi-frown. That is usually followed by "Why would you want to do that?" or something along those lines. Then, of course, I have to explain why working with and understanding older people is so important.

Since I was very young, I have had an affinity for persons older than me. Why? That's a good question, and I guess the best answer is probably that I spent a lot of time with my grandparents. In interacting with them, I was able to see what older people were really like. As I've grown older, I've seen how the world around me reacts to senior citizens and have seen the various stereotypes and ideas about these older people, many of which are not true. The list is endless, from the classic stereotype of the "grumpy old man" or the "mean old bitty" to the slowdriving 80-year-old. Other stereotypes, like assuming most older persons end up in nursing homes and are always chronically ill and in pain have also permeated society. However, a lot of education is needed to correct these sorts of ideas and return the view of older citizens to the truth.

One of my classmates on this day, and my good friend, after looking at the presentation slides, was not very happy about discussing older people. She informed everyone in the class that older people are grumpy and gross and that she just did not see why she needed to learn about them. She informed us that she would only be taking care of "pregnant women and babies," so old people did not apply to her. Interestingly, she got a shock that week during clinical.

While the details are a bit sketchy since I was not there, this student, who shall remain nameless, ended up taking care of an older adult patient that had broken her hip. The patient was, according to my friend, a "spitfire." She was the classic, stereotyped older adult female: wrinkles, "grey" hair, eye glasses. She walked several miles every day, went on vacations with her grandchildren all the time, and also enjoyed being in several clubs. When the student asked this patient what her concerns about the next few weeks were, the patient asked something along the lines of, "Well, I really want to know when I can have sex again. When will my hip be well enough again?" And did I mention that this patient was single?

To hear my friend, the same friend that had a very set vision of older adults in her mind, tell this story was comical. Not only could the student not believe that this patient was having sex, but she also could not believe that she was *single* and having sex. How dare this older adult express her sexuality!

That clinical day, this student's mind was opened up just a bit. She learned a couple lessons. First, patients are not always what they may seem to be based on certain stereotypes and, second, it is important to talk with patients and find out what their concerns are because those concerns may just surprise you. Further, what is learned from talking with the patient will largely influence what sort of teaching the nurse needs to do.

Interestingly, a long-standing stereotype has been that older people either a) don't want to have sex or b) can't have sex for one reason or another. However, both of these ideas are incorrect (though some minor elements may be true). Other than for "fun," why are sexual relations even important in older adulthood? The reason it is important is that it helps to improve intimacy, closeness and touch in the lives of all persons, including older adults. The warm feelings and psychological changes (through the release of various chemicals in the brain) help make people feel better and, in turn, live higher quality lives. Furthermore, looking at the more obvious, it can be a source of physical activity. Sexual relations is actually an integral part of life, and sexual feelings frequently remain into old age (see for example Lenahan & Ellwood, 2004). One study by Bretcheider and McCoy (1988), which is admittedly slightly dated (but very informative), took a look at the sex lives of older persons between 80 and 102 years old. (How would you like to have been those researchers?) This research found that 62% of the men studied and 30% of the women reported that they were currently sexually active; 83% of the men and 64% of the women reported that they had engaged in some other type of "sexual expression," such as self-pleasuring (masturbation).

On a quick note to explain the physiology behind sexuality and aging, as women reach menopause at between 40 and 55 (approximately), female reproductive hormones (estrogens in particular) decline significantly; while one might think that this would cause a decreased libido, in fact, it does not, as it is believed that some adrenal sex steroids are able to maintain sexual desire in females (see for example Tortora & Derrickson, 2009). For males, similar is true. Sperm production decreases significantly between 60 and 80, but there may still be significant amounts of sperm production well past 80, and certain hormones or steroids in the body compensate for any lost testosterone due to aging. Their sex drive continues and is not significantly impacted.

But why is it even important for nurses to understand a patient's sexual activity, especially when the patient is an older adult? The same risks present in younger persons having intercourse is still intact in older age (minus the risk of having unwanted children, in most cases). Because older adults feel that they cannot get pregnant or because they may not understand the issues behind sexually transmitted diseases (STDs) and sexually transmitted infections (STIs), they may not use barrier protection. Barrier protection includes tools like condoms and diaphragms. Furthermore, because of weakened immune systems, older adults may be more at risk for STIs and STDs, as their bodies are not as good at fighting off pathogens, or infections agents, such as bacteria or viruses. There is some debate on the use of the term STD vs. STI, but, in general, STDs are those that cause a disease, such as Human Immunodeficiency Virus (HIV). STIs, on the other hand are not long-term diseases but rather infections that can generally be treated, like chlamydia or gonorrhea.

STDs and STIs in the older population are actually not uncommon, as many older people do not practice safe sex because they do not realize they are at risk or have not been educated properly about protection (see for example Morley & Tariq, 2003 and Wooten-Bielski, 1999). If you need statistical proof, between 2005 and 2009, the number of persons over 55 with chlamydia increased 41 %, and the Centers for Disease Control and Prevention reports that about 10% of new AIDS cases in the United States appear in those over the age of 50 (see Johns Hopkins, 2011). Furthermore, one study that looked at 2,000 people found that about 66% of the men and women in the study had not used a condom in their last sexual encounter. Additionally, of those encounters, 43% of men reported that their sexual partner was not a spouse. Just as sex education is important for young people (and at an even earlier age than in the past), sex education is important for older adults, too. Some senior citizens may never have had any formal sexual education in school, so they are especially in need of proper education. So, as the nurse, it would be important to teach the older adult about safe sex, even though it might be a rather uncomfortable conversation.

Other issues applicable to nursing can also be troublesome in regard to sexuality in seniors. When should a person be stopped from having sexual relations? Should nursing homes and other institutions prohibit sexual relations in the facility if it is a natural part of human interaction? What if a person with moderate or even severe dementia makes the decision to have sex? Is that okay, even though he or she may not be able to cognitively make sense of what is happening? What if this person sexually assaults a staff member or another resident but does not think it is sexual assault because of the dementia? As illustrated, certain ethical/moral dilemmas can arise when libido and cognition face off against one another, and nurses must be able to wrap their minds around these issues as well.

Even though this chapter spent a good deal of time discussing older adults and their activity in the bedroom, the end message is fairly simple: no patient is as simple or as straightforward as he or she may seem, and stereotypes must be thrown out the door, especially in nursing. Further, no issue is ever simple. Sexuality in older adults quickly turns into an ethical dilemma, and misunderstandings of health care providers can lead to inadequate care for older adults.

Ch. 27:
Understanding the Homeless

During community health, we spent time working with several community organizations and institutions. One such institution was a local homeless shelter that was only open during the day. Because this was a short experience, our major goal was to get to know some of the clients that used the shelter and to try to learn more about their lives. We didn't need to come up with care plans and so forth; we only needed to make meaningful conversation.

When I first arrived at the shelter, I saw a room full of vulnerable people (minus some of the people in there that just use the shelter for a social outlet). I meandered over to one of my classmates Lisa, who was already there and working at the coffee area. She had been there since 7:00 AM and said her morning had been pretty uneventful, other than a couple of gentlemen trying to hit on her.

After seeing how she was, I made my first "move." I spotted an older man, Ed, sitting at a table by himself and took a seat next to him. I simply asked, "Hi, how's it going?" He responded with a "hello," and after a couple minutes he asked where I was from. I explained to him that I was a nursing student. He then began talking about his work as a handyman that he does with his friend. He talked about not being able to ever do anything "good enough" for his friend, and I shared the sentiment that sometimes it seems like whatever a person does, sometimes it just seems like some people cannot be made happy. We then began talking about the nurse practitioner, as he was waiting to see her. He seemed to appreciate the service provided him.

He left, and I then met Remmy, whom I eventually had contact with again later in the day. Remmy had a very interesting history. He actually worked as an LPN for a few years. Remmy and I had a good conversation about common sense. He discussed those that use drugs and alcohol and how they have no common sense. (I couldn't ascertain whether or not he had personal experience with "common sense" or not.) Additionally I discussed my feelings about the homeless population, as he was interested in what I thought. I told him that I felt they were a worthy population, just like middle class and rich people. He and I discussed the fact that a lot of the homeless think that people "on the other side of the fence" think that they can snap their fingers and solve the homeless problem. He was delighted to hear what I had to say. Remmy and I continued on, talking about the coffee. He also talked to me about some of the other people at the shelter. When I got ready to leave later in the day, Remmy was leaning up against the side of the building, so I visited with him for a few minutes. He told me I need to get a job at the shelter and work with the people there, and I explained to him my situation but suggested I'd be back another day. I did in fact visit the shelter several other times.

As people started to return from lunch that they had at a soup kitchen down the block, I found another "opportunity." I sat down next to perhaps the most interesting person of the day, Lilly. Lilly enjoyed art and enjoyed going to many of the art festivals in town. We talked about all kinds of art, and then we arrived at the topic of music. For about 30 minutes, we did nothing but talk about Bob Dylan, Jimmy Buffet, The Beatles, the Bee Gees, Benny Goodman, and many more. I actually liked a lot of the music she did, so we talked about various songs and styles. Also, Lilly talked about being a "ringer" for the Salvation Army. She loved that job because she got to see her cousins and also was able to see old high school friends going in and out of stores. In fact, she talked about running into a boy that she had a crush on in high school. She said she was the geek and awkward person in high school, and he was the stud. Now, however, she informed me the roles had changed. She said she was now the popular one and that she had the looks and he was simply "ugly."

Then there was Kendra. She was in her 70s and was sexually assaulted a few years ago; she shared with me how much one of the local health centers had helped her after the attack. Prior to getting help, she told me how much her self-respect had suffered. She talked about singing in the choir at church and feeling that everyone was staring at her because she had such a feeling of guilt. She talked about how it tore her apart and how she felt like a worthless person that deserved to be raped. She did, though, say she had gotten much better because of the help she received from the health center she visited. I wish I could have had more time with Kendra, but I had to leave to return to the health clinic for post-conference.

One of the biggest take-home points I left with was that these homeless individuals were human beings. Many of them were intelligent – in one way or another – and many had just fallen on hard times. Several of the individuals my classmates and I met had received some level of education and had even had decent jobs. By and large, these individuals had made one or two major mistakes in life which had changed their trajectory from a wonderful, successful life to a life on the streets. It was certainly a humbling and eye-opening experience.

Ch. 28:
Home Visits and
"Operation Find-A-Bed"

By some miracle, nursing school was coming to an end. In just about three and a half months, I would be done with nursing school. All that stood in my way was Intercultural Communication, Principles of Teaching and Learning, Transitions to Professional Nursing, and . . . Community Health. By this semester, we were left with 24 students, and, essentially, we just needed to survive until May.

Community health was unlike any other rotation we completed in nursing school. For this semester, we focused on the outpatient setting, and we would be making home visits. Home visits created a lot of anxiety for the students in my class. What would it be like to step into patients' homes – their "turf?"

We were used to being in control, as much as we were used to having clinical in the hospital setting. The hospital was a familiar place, and we had all of the resources around us necessary to provide care (and help us if we needed it). In community, however, the level of autonomy skyrocketed. While we still had clinical "groups," each student was assigned two or three patients for the entire semester, and we would spend several months getting to know these patients and working towards several goals, all realated to improving their health. Each student in the group went to a different patient home, and our instructor, Dr. Weed, was essentially "on call," in case one of us needed assistance. However, that assistance could take a while to get there, if Dr. Weed was across town with another student.

This semester, I was assigned two patients. While I would tell the story of both sets of patients, for one of the patients, the story – even with details changed – would be too obvious, and I'm afraid I could compromise the patient's confidentiality. Thus, I will just tell the story of one of my patients for the semester.

Our "home base" for the semester would be a community health clinic, and the patients we were assigned to were generally patients of this clinic. Tuesday, we met at the clinic for orientation, and Thursday, we found out exactly which patients we would be assigned to. As I walked into the clinic on Thursday morning, I considered the possibilities in my head. I knew I would have two patients to work with, but I really had no idea what to expect – these patients could have any problem(s) and medical diagnoses they were dealing with, and they could live anywhere in the entire city. Would I be assigned a young adult with terminal cancer? What about an older adult who needed close diabetes management? Or would it be a newborn infant who wasn't gaining weight? The options were truly endless, and I didn't know what to expect. All of this uncertainty was making me nervous, and I was ready to find out my assignment.

I made my way down the hallway to the large conference room. Each morning when we met for pre-conference, I always felt like I was at a meeting with executives, ready to discuss business strategy, rather than discuss our patients, simply because the table was a "classic" boardroom table, and the chairs were executive-worthy office chairs – very comfortable (in fact, occasionally too comfortable in the early morning hours). Dr. Weed was already there, busy rummaging through several files on the desk, and I said good morning to a few of my classmates, including Monica, who looked like she was about ready to vomit. "What if I get a patient that lives in a really bad part of town?" she asked. "I'm not about to get shot after having been through 7 semesters of nursing school."

After the usual pleasantries, Dr. Weed informed us that she would be giving us our patients' names and addresses, and we would need to look up their phone numbers. Our major task for the day would be twofold – first, we needed to make contact with both of our patients either by phone or by home visit, and we would also need to collect relevant data from the patients' files.

"Here we go," I thought to myself. "Let's make this good, Dr. Weed."

As luck would have it, or not have it, I was last out of the other nine students in room. I had been listening to Dr. Weed go through the various patients with my classmates – talking about patients with just about every problem under the sun, from spina bifida to end-stage renal disease to malnutrition. It was finally my turn.

"Oh, okay. So John, you actually get what I'll call a bargain," Dr. Weed began.

I knew there was no way this was actually going to be a bargain. I had the sneaking suspicion that "bargain" was code for "more work," and more work was the last thing I wanted for my last semester of nursing school when I had hoped for at least some level of sanity and time of my own.

"You'll get your pediatric patient, too (the patient I'm going to leave out of my discussion here), but you're actually going to get a married couple as your 'patient.' Dr. Silvia (the clinic's main physician) informed me that both of these individuals need follow-up care at home, and so you'll have the opportunity to care for both of these patients," she explained. "Their names are Emory and Deena Mulgrew – 72 and 74 years old."

Several of my classmates had patients that were married, but their only patient was one member of the dyad – not both.

"Oh greeeeat... the 'opporunity'," I thought to myself. Of course, on the outside, I managed a half smile and just responded, "Oh, interesting. That should be different." That's about all I had at that moment. It's not that I did not want to care for patients. I was just tired and needed a break. An extra patient meant an extra care plan, extra drug cards, extra progress notes, extra preparation time, and so forth. I felt it was a bit unfair that I would have a total of three patients, while my classmates would only have two, but I took it in stride, and over the semester, Dr. Weed actually allowed me to be a bit more flexible with my schedule and due dates for assignments, given I had an increased workload.

After I finished getting my pediatric patient assignment, I headed for the nursing station to start gathering some patient information and to find the phone numbers for both of my patients. I found out that, essentially, Mr. Mulgrew had fairly advanced diabetes and suffered from a loss of sensation in his lower extremities because of it, termed diabetic neuropathy. He had a recent wound on his foot that needed monitoring so that it would heal and not get worse. Mrs. Mulgrew was suffering from COPD, making it very difficult for her to breathe effectively. She had to wear oxygen at all times, in fact. I was already brainstorming care plan possibilities.

It was then time to make the call. What would they say when I called? Would they think this was some sort of scam?

I dialed the number. I head a "ring…" followed by a "ring…" followed by another "ring…" They didn't answer. I tried one more time twenty minutes later, but there was still no answer. I explained the situation to Dr. Weed, and she suggested I make a home visit the following Tuesday to try to make contact with them, if they didn't answer their phone again that day.

Of course, there was still no answer on Tuesday, and so it was off to make an unannounced home visit. Dr. Weed said that she would go with me, just in case they were leary of a random student showing up at their doorstep, and she even offered to drive. It was February, and so the drive over was no easy feat – we were lucky enough to have to put up with about six inches of snow, but I was certainly glad to be the passenger and not the driver in this weather. After a 20 minute drive that should have taken us about five minutes, we finally arrived at the Mulgrew residence. The "residence" was actually a one-bedroom apartment in a seven story apartment building, which I would later find out was reserved for low-income seniors.

"Welcome to Golden Towers," the sign read as we walked in the lobby area. The building had an old, musty smell – a cross between stale cigarettes from a decade before and mold. We looked for an elevator, but we soon received a surprise. The elevator had stopped working that morning, according to one of the older adults milling about the lobby. According to the sign on the elevator door, it would be fixed "soon." Accordingly, it was time for some cardio – the stairs. We trudged up the stairwell, moving quicker than normal, given that the stairwell was especially cold.

We finally made it to the Mulgrew apartment – #702. The door was flimsy-looking and light brown with multiple nicks in it. It didn't look like it had been painted in years.

I knocked on the door a couple times, fairly lightly, but there was no response. Then, Dr. Weed, with a flurry of energy, knocked, no – pounded – on the door with her hand. She did not mess around when it came to knocking on doors, I found out. She wanted to be sure anyone within a 10-block radius would know we were at the door.

I heard the slow pitter-patter of feet heading toward the door, and slowly, the door creaked open. An elderly looking gentleman opened the door about two inches – just far enough to peer out to see who was on the other side of the door. As Dr. Weed and I were dressed in our nice clothes and a white lab coat, he apparently could tell we meant him no harm.

"Hello," he said. "Can I help ya?"

I wanted to respond, but Dr. Weed jumped in first. "I'm Marilyn Weed, a nursing professor with the school of nursing, and this is John, a nursing student. We are working at the community health clinic with Dr. Silvia this semester, and she thought that you and your wife might be able to benefit from our free services this semester."

"Hmm. She didn't say anything about it at our last appointment, but if she thinks we need it, I guess maybe we can. I'll need to talk with the wife and see what she thinks. What would all this entail?" he questioned us, still sounding suspicious.

Dr. Weed again responded, "Essentially John would be bringing the doctor's office to you each week. He would stop by either Tuesday or Thursday morning at a time of your choice and would take your blood pressure, see how you are feeling, and work on some health goals with you."

"Doesn't sound like a bad deal. But you say it's free?" Mr. Mulgrew asked.

"Absolutely free. It's part of John's nursing eduation," Dr. Weed responded.

During this entire interaction, I was essentially left standing there, smiling and nodding. I never did feel that comfortable talking to patients in front of faculty members, but in this case, I didn't need to do any talking, since Dr. Weed was taking care of it all.

Mr. Mulgrew dismissed himself temporarily to go talk with his wife, and she gave us the okay. As they were getting ready to leave for a church function, they couldn't meet with me that morning, but I set up a meeting for the coming Thursday.

I showed up about 10 minutes early – 9:20 AM. I wasn't quite sure how this meeting would go. I still questioned what it would be like to walk into someone's home – their castle, not mine.

I knocked on the door, using more force this time than I had during our previous visit. Again, I heard the slow pitter patter of feet across the floor. Mr. Mulgrew opened the door. "Oh good morning," he said politely. "Come on in."

I made my way into the home with my nursing bag on my shoulder. This bag contained all the essentials – manual blood pressure cuff, thermometer, stethoscope, pen light, and so forth.

As I scanned the room, I quickly found out that the Mulgrews had a very small apartment. Their kitchen, dining room and living area were essentially all one, and only one other door was visible, which I assumed was the bedroom. The furniture appeared to be from about 1960, and the musty smell in the apartment was even worse than what we encountered in the lobby area. Stacks of paper lay strewn about, and the corners of the apartment were filled with cobwebs. Several old McDonalds value meal cups were stacked next to the recliner, and I could see several crumpled up Burger King bags littering the dining room table.

"My goodness, these poor people," I thought to myself. "I wonder how long they've lived this way."

"So sorry things are messy around here, John," Mrs. Mulgrew apologized. "I just don't have any energy to do any cleaning anymore. This is about all we can manage."

I introduced myself fully, and gave them a bit of background, reviewing what Dr. Weed had mentioned at our first meeting.

"Well, Mr. and Mrs. Mulgrew (I had a bad habit of starting sentences with "well) I'd like to get to know you both a little better today and find out what I can do to assist you – find out your priorities and ideas. Then, next week, maybe we can start achieving some goals," I suggested with a smile.

"Oh, you don't have to call us Mr. and Mrs. – please, if we are going to be together, you might as well call us Emory and Deena," Mrs. Mulgrew insisted with a heartwarming smile. Emory and Deena together seemed so happy. Even in such a dim home environment, the couple seemed to enjoy life and each other. The walls were dotted with pictures of what I assumed to be family and friends. "This is our family," Deena said, handing me a 5 x 7 picture with about 15 people in it – Emory and Deena at the center, sitting in chairs. "We don't see them too often because they live hours away, but we sure enjoy family."

"What a wonderful picture," I responded. After a little bit more getting to know each other, I began to delve into the couple's health. "So if there were one thing you could improve in regard to your helath this semester, what would it be?" I asked. While I had some of my own priorities in mind, having already practically stalked them by reading through countless MD progress notes and their entire health histories, I always (and still do) felt it was very important to get to know my patients' priorities – what they think is relevant. If I only ever did what I thought was best, that could have created conflict and also gotten us nowhere.

Emory responded first, "Well, really, I feel pretty good, but the missus, she's always short of breath and never seems to have any energy." This became a common theme – not shortness of breath but the fact that Emory never wanted me to focus on him. He always wanted my focus to be on his wife.

"Oh, I'm doing alright," Deena responded. "I just have a little trouble now and then, but I don't feel *that* bad." This also became a common theme – Deena downplaying the severity of her symptoms or insisting that she was "doing alright."

After a little additional discussion, I asked if it would be okay to perform a full head-to-toe assessment on both of them so that I could get an idea where they were at. I also needed to take a peak at Mr. Mulgrew's foot wound. They were both willing to allow me to assess them, and so I did, systematically moving from head to toe. All-in-all they seemed to be healthy overall, except for Deena's lungs, which were extremely over-inflated and sounded terrible – full of wheezes. "How would you compare your breathing today to a month ago?" I asked.

"Well, I'd say it's about the same. Not that much worse," Deena responded.

"Hmm," I thought. "Not *that* much worse. Her response told me it was worse, but I wasn't sure just how much worse."

It was about time for me to go so that I could make it back to the health clinic in time for post-conference, so I said my goodbyes and asked if there was anything specific they needed me to do prior to the next visit, which they declined.

I also wanted to take another look at Deena's medical record to see when her last diagnostic tests were – blood and x-ray – so that I could see whether repeat testing might be considered, before going to Dr. Silvia. As it turned out, her tests had been on the Friday before my visit, and they were stable as compared with her previous exams.

I returned the following week with some ideas in hand. For Mr. Mulgrew, my priority would be helping his foot wound to heal and controlling his diabetes more effectively. His blood sugars had been running in the high 100s to low 200s for months, and the higher glucose levels only encouraged bacterial growth in his foot and made it more difficult for the wound to heal. As for Mrs. Mulgrew, my priority was to prevent decline in her respiratory status and work on ways to help her breathe a bit easier.

After changing Emory's foot wound dressing, which was actually healing nicely, I asked him how often he checked his blood sugars.

"Oh, maybe once a week," he responded. "It's always high, so I never really feel the need to check it, plus those strips for the machine are so dang expensive."

This problem was common. Strips for glucose meters were quite expensive, and from Mr. Mulgrew's perspective, only checking blood sugars once or so per week seemed logical. This day, we spent most of the time discussing the importance of glucose monitoring and the effect of diet on the glucose level. While Mr. Mulgrew understood that sugar was bad for him, he had a hard time understanding how some foods (really every food) are transformed into glucose eventually.

"I don't add any sugar, but my sugar level is always high for some reason," he explained to me. "I try, but it's still high."

After futher investigation, it became obvious that he was eating other foods high in protein and carbohydrates, and reading food labels was a bit of a chore for him. I would add nutrition label reading to my plan for the following week, I thought to myself.

I then turned my attention to Mrs. Mulgrew. "How are you feeling this week," I asked her.

"Oh, just a little punky," she answered me. "What do you mean by punky?" I asked. I hadn't noticed it before, but Deena looked very tired today. She was pale, and her eyes seemed like they wanted to retreat into her skull.

"I've just had a little more fatigue lately," she responded.

"Anything else going on?" I asked. "What about any worsening shortness of breath? Any chest pain?"

"No. Well, I don't know. Maybe it's a little worse. And I've just had a bit of chest pain but only when I cough or breathe deeply. I've developed this cough that seems to come and go."

I ran through all of the typical respiratory and cardiovascular symptom questions with her, trying to get a better idea what was going on. "Is anything coming up when you cough – any mucous?" I continued.

"Not really," she responded.

"Well, let's take a listen to your lungs. I'll also check your vital signs and see if I find anything abnormal," I said. I also text messaged Dr. Weed and asked her if she could bring the portable pulse oximeter machine to me. Essentially, this machine helped to measure the oxygen level in the blood, and I wanted to find out how well Mrs. Mulgrew was oxygenated. Additionally, I wanted Dr. Weed to take a look at Deena to see what she thought.

After further assessment, it became fairly obvious something was going on. Deena's temperature was 99.7

Fahrenheit – a low grade fever, and her lungs sounded like there was some consolidion – a buildup of material (usually mucous) in the lungs. Her oxygen level was also a bit lower than what she normally achieved at her office visits, but it was still in the "normal" range. At this point, I was suspicious for a lung infection – some type of pneumonia. Dr. Weed concurred, and I explained my plan to the couple.

"I'm going to run back to the clinic and chat with Dr. Silvia to let her know what's going on. She might want to do some tests and make sure you're not getting sick," I explained. Of course, I knew that testing was almost a certainty, but I didn't want to get Mr. or Mrs. Mulgrew too upset.

Sure enough, after explaining the situation to Dr. Silvia, she ordered some blood work and a chest x-ray, and so I gave the Mulgrews a call to update them and instruct them to come to the clinic for the testing. "Do you think it's pneumonia? Will she need medicine?" Emory asked me.

I answered him honestly and said, "I don't know for sure. We will know more after the tests," I answered. That was about the best I could do at the time.

Sure enough, the x-ray came back showing an area in the lung that was full of mucous, and the lab work revealed that there was likely an infectious process going on, since the white blood cell count was high. These results didn't come back until later in the afternoon on Tuesday, however, so I didn't find out about them until Thursday morning. Thursday morning I also found out that Dr. Silvia had admitted Deena to the local hospital with pneumonia.

We followed our patients, so whether they were at home, in the hospital or in some other setting, it was our job to go there. Thus, while I did not have a scheduled appointment with the couple until the following week, given Mrs. Mulgrew's illness, I wanted to check up on them that day and so I headed for the hospital after pre-conference.

I was surprised to learn that Mrs. Mulgrew had been admitted to the intensive care unit after first being in the general medical unit. I made my way up to the 5th floor and walked to the ICU. It seemed very busy that day, but in very little time, I was able to track down Deena's nurse to try and get an update. According to Deena's nurse, she had been on the general unit when her blood pressure began to creep down, and some blood work revealed she had a systemic infection – sepsis. Now, the priority was keeping her blood pressure up and treating the infection with multiple IV antibiotics. She was on continuous fluids to help with the blood pressure, along with an additional IV medication. For the moment, Mrs. Mulgrew was stable, but I was afraid things could get worse, especially because of her existing severe COPD.

After the update from the nurse, I went to go see Mr. and Mrs. Mulgrew. I found room 8 and peaked my head around the glass door that led to the room. Mrs. Mulgrew was sound asleep, but even in rest, she looked as if she were worn out. Her skin was as pale as ever, and she had several IV tubes running into her body. Mr. Mulgrew sat in the corner with his cane at his side.

"Oh, goodness John. I didn't know she was *this* sick," said Mr. Mulgrew in a rather exhausted tone. "I just hope she makes it. I – I can't continue on without her, I know that," he noted, beginning to tear up.

I walked over to Mr. Mulgrew and shook his hand, assuring him that his wife was being well taken care of and that she was being treated as effectively as she could be at the time.

"Do you think that she will make it," he asked me.

I knew this question was coming, and I felt conflicted in how to answer it. I was dreading having to answer. We were taught never to lie to patients or to give them any false hope, but at the same time, I saw the anxiety in Mr. Mulgrew's eyes. If I told the absolute truth – that there was a chance she could die anytime – it would have crushed him, but if I insisted that she would pull through, this could have given him a false sense of security. In the end, I settled for an answer somewhere in between. "To be honest, Emory," I started, "I don't know the answer to that. Certainly with all of the medications she is getting and the high level of care, she is being given the best chance, but sepsis is scary, and I can't promise you you're out of the woods. Basically, it's a game of wait and see."

While this answer didn't destroy Emory, it did cause him to again ponder the possibility that his beloved wife could be taken from him at any moment. "Well, alright then," was his only response.

I stayed with Emory while Deena slept and talked for about twenty more minutes, answering questions he had about the medications and what to expect in the coming days. I honestly did not know what would happen.

When I returned the following Tuesday to check up on the couple, things were looking much better. Mrs. Mulgrew was out of the ICU and was on a general medical unit now – only receiving two antibiotics but no fluids or additional treatment for her blood pressure. Of course, when I entered the hospital room, I knew exactly where to find Emory. He was sitting in the corner, taking a bite of his donut. (Given his diabetes, a donut was clearly not a good breakfast choice, but I didn't have the heart to say anything to him about it at that point.)

"Good morning," I said. "It looks like things are on their way up now."

"Yes, finally," Emory responded.

"Thanks for coming to see me," Deena added. Of course, this was part of my job as a student nurse, but that did not matter to Deena – she was appreciative of me even if I *had* to do what I was doing.

We discussed what would happen once Deena got back home, and I then brought up diabetes control with Emory. We talked about reading food labels, and I had a few items from the nutrition room at the hospital to demonstrate with. Emory picked right up on interpreting these labels and admitted he had not really read the labels much previously, though he assured me he would start doing so. We also discussed a goal number of carbohydrates for him to eat in a day.

A short while later, I dismissed myself, as I had another appointment with my pediatric patient. My plan was to come back Thursday for an update.

I returned Thursday and found out that Deena would be going home, most likely, on Friday. She would be switching over to oral antibiotic pills instead of the IV. This was fantastic news, and I was relieved. At the outset, I wasn't really sure whether Mrs. Mulgrew would ever make it out of the hospital, but luckily, she had done exceptionally well.

I continued to make house calls for several weeks. We focused on various topics, such as medication adherence strategies for both of them, as it had become clear to me that they did not always take medications correctly, and I also tracked Mr. Mulgrew's foot wound progress, along with Mrs. Mulgrew's post-hospitalization progress. Both of them had high blood pressure, and they had an automatic blood pressure machine at home, but it had no batteries, so I purchased some batteries for the machine. Working together, we created a log for both of their blood pressures and Mr. Mulgrew's blood sugars. We made good progress throughout the semester.

However, even with the progress that was made, one lingering issue stood in the way – a queen-size bed. The couple had not had a bed to sleep on for years. One day, after checking vital signs, I had brought up the topic of sleep and asked them how well they slept at night.

"Um, well we actually sleep here, in these chairs," Deena answered me. "We don't really have a bed."

There was no "really." She could have just said, "We don't have a bed." "How in the world do they manage?" I thought to myself.

"Would you like to have a bed?" I asked them.

"Well it sure would be nice, but we just don't have the money for it, and we get along okay in our chairs," Emory insisted.

This was not a good enough answer for me. I decided it would be my mission to get the couple a queen-size bed that they could sleep in. But how would I go about this task?

There were only two weeks of clinical left, so I knew I needed to move quickly. I enlisted the help of another classmate, Lisa, after receiving the go-ahead from Dr. Weed. From this point forward, Lisa and I embarked on what we liked to call "Operation Find-A-Bed."

Dr. Weed provided us with a list of community agencies that might be able to help, and the hunting began. Lisa and I spent the next three clinical days scouring the city, trying to find the perfect bed.

On Tuesday, we arrived at the 18th Street Mission at 5:30 AM. The doors opened at 8:00 AM, but in order to be in the front of the line and to get the "good stuff," like a bed, we had to get there early. When we arrived, there were already three people ahead of us. Everyone looked at us like we had ten eyes. Lisa and I were both dressed in our uniforms with our white lab coats on. The people there weren't sure what we were doing. They eyed us rather suspiciously, and I'm pretty sure they thought we were there to ask questions, rather than try to get our hands on some items.

The mission was located in one of the worst neighborhoods of Decatur, and Lisa and I both felt uncomfortable, though by our last semester in nursing school, we had been in some pretty rough situations. Two and a half hours later, the mission opened. We were both out of place. The other people there (about thirty by that point) all seemed to know what to do – go inside, get a number, fill out a request form for what was needed and why. Our number was 322.

"Number 322," one of the volunteers called.

We made our way up to the desk, but the volunteer informed us that there were "no beds today" and that we could "come back Thursday."

"Wonderful," I thought to myself. The adventure continues. But Lisa had an idea.

"How much money do you have in your pocket?" Lisa asked me. "Right now, probably 20 or 30 bucks," I responded.

"I have probably about the same amount," Lisa commented. "Maybe we could go thrift shopping."

"Thrift shopping!" I thought to myself. This would be a game changer. Amusingly, the song "Thrift Shop" by Macklemore and Ryan Lewis was popular at the time, and both Lisa and I laughed to ourselves about that as we got into my Ford Ranger to begin the thrift shopping expedition. It didn't take long to hear the song on the radio, either. We were on our way to our first stop when the song came on, and both of us laughed, rolled down the windows, and turned up the volume.

We had consulted Google for the nearest thrift shops and found out one was located at the corner of 20th and Miller St. This was to be our first stop. The building looked more like an old car shop than a thrift shop. One wall of the stablishment was old garage doors, and the other was just plywood. "Look!" I said to Lisa, pointing at a bed in the corner.

We walked over to the bed and inspected the item.

"It's only $15," Lisa commented. "It's so cheap."

The mattress didn't look terrible, and the bed frame appeared to be in good shape. However, when we turned the mattress over, we discovered why the set was only $15. There were several large stains on it, and neither of us were certain what the stains were from – it could have been anything, really.

Disappointed, we set out for the next thrift shop. The cycle seemed to repeat itself. We went to four thrift shops in total that day, and we met four equally disgusting mattresses.

We returned to post-conference that day feeling defeated, but, as it turned out, it was a good thing that we hadn't found a mattress and frame. After we explained our morning to Dr. Weed, she chuckled and informed us that it was good we hadn't found a mattress. "It's actually illegal for them to sell used mattresses," she explained. "Maybe we can find a mattress frame for them and then work another way to get them a mattress."

This seemed like a reasonable plan to me, and Lisa agreed. We had dodged a bullet, luckily. Our plan was to return to one of the thrift shops where we had located a frame, and we did so the following week.

In the end, we were able to secure a frame for the Mulgrews, and after they received the frame, their family members actually went together to buy them a queen-size mattress. While the mattress had not been delivered by the time the semester was over, both of the Mulgrews assured Lisa and me that they were extremely grateful to us.

"I told you I'd find you a bed," I noted, "I guess we got halfway there with the frame."

"You have helped us so much these last few months," Deena noted. "Who knows what we would have done without you."

Looking back on the semester, community health was indeed much different than any other semester. We were able to spend over three months with the same patients, and we had much more autonomy. Also, given the extended time we had to work with the patients, I felt like I was actually able to make significant impact on my patients' lives.

PART VII: GRADUATION

Ch. 29:
The Exit Interview

Renowned fantasy writer, Ray Bradbury, once said, "I spent three days a week for 10 years educating myself in the public library, and it's better than college. People should educate themselves – you can get a complete education for no money."

While I certainly understand his sentiment, with apologies to Mr. Bradbury, it would have been impossible for me to learn the amount of information that I did and experience the situations and emotions that I did without college – without four years of intense education and countless hours spent with patients inside and outside of the hospital. I was able to put theory to practice and expand my understanding of not only nursing but also humanity as a whole.

As part of our requirements for graduation, we were all mandated to meet with our academic advisors for what was termed an "exit interview." During this interview we would talk about several things, including our reflections on our years in nursing school, employment opportunities for after graduation (which was an ongoing discussion with our advisors), and plans for studying for the national licensing exam – the NCLEX. After all, if we could not pass our licensing exam, we wouldn't practice as nurses.

I set up an exit interview meeting with my academic advisor, Dr. Sheryl Samuelson, PhD, RN, for a Tuesday afternoon – 2:00 PM. These interviews were expected to take about 20 to 30 minutes, but I knew better. I planned on spending at least an hour in her office.

My friends and I all had different levels of relationships with our academic advisors, and some had closer ties than others. For me, meeting with my advisor had become commonplace. Truthfully, we rarely had official "meetings." I would drop in several times a week just to "shoot the breeze" and share thoughts. While to the outside observer our conversations likely seemed to be just random discussions with a lot of laughs and hollering intermixed, quite honestly, we had very deep conversations and reflected frequently on current events. We contemplated the meaning of life, sure, and we discussed the latest fate of the Green Bay Packers (for her sake), but we also talked about serious topics like reducing patient suicides in-hospital, improving outcomes of patients with heart failure, minimizing restraint use in hospitals, developing appropriate curriculum for nursing students, working in the "real world," and many more. We also discussed my future – where I would pursue further education, what job I would take upon graduation, and so forth. Heck, we even went on several "road trips" together to academic events and research presentations, including traveling to Rush University in Chicago, the American Psychiatric Nurses Association annual conference in Louisville, Kentucky, and the Glore Psychiatric Museum in St. Joseph, Missouri. Starting my freshman year, I had developed close ties with Dr. Samuelson when we began a research project together. She was and is my mentor, and I have learned a great deal from her. In fact, when it came time to select an academic advisor for my graduate program, I selected her.

At about 1:45 PM, I left my residence hall room and headed for the nursing building. I wondered what I would say during the meeting. I hadn't really thought too much about it, mainly because I had been in a flurry, trying to finish several projects for the end of the semester.

I walked into the School of Nursing office and headed to the back corner, where Dr. Samuelson's office was located. I poked my head around the door and gave her a smile; she was just finishing typing an email and invited me to come on in and have a seat.

My eyes wandered around her office while I waited. In the corner to my right, I saw two posters wrapped up and tucked neatly in a box. Both of these posters I had played a role in during my tenure as an undergraduate. On the wall opposite the posters was a large poster-sized picture of a piece of embroidery created by a patient with schizophrenia. This happened to be a piece of embroidery that Dr. Samuelson, another student, and I had researched during my freshman and sophomore year. On the bulletin board above her computer, I noted a newspaper article, tacked up very neatly. The title read "John Blakeman recognized for research work in nursing." Her entire office seemed to be a summary of my years in nursing school. Seeing those items brought back some tremendous memories. I chuckled out loud, thinking of some of these memories.

"What's so funny?" Dr. Samuelson asked me.

"Oh, I was just thinking about how far I've come," I responded. "Can you believe it? I remember freshman year talking about having four years to accomplish all kinds of goals. Here we are – four years later. It's really hard to believe."

"Well, it certainly has gone by quickly," she answered. "You're not done yet, though. You have more work to do," she commented with a smile.

I knew what she meant. At that point, she knew I was planning on earning my Master of Science in Nursing degree and most likely going on to obtain a doctorate.

"Very true," I noted.

We then spent about twenty minutes discussing the necessary items for the exit interview – my studying plans to prepare for my national licensing exam, my finalized post-graduation job, and so on. But then came the fun part.

This is how most of our meetings went. The first portion of the meeting, we would accomplish our goal for the day. Then, we would spend the rest of the time sharing stories and bouncing ideas off of one another.

"So what is your biggest revelation from the last few years? What stuck out to you the most?" Dr. Samuelson asked. She had a habit of asking a lot of emotion-driven questions and always wanted to hear my perspective. This was likely partly due to the fact she had spent years in the psychiatric-mental health nursing field and at one point was a clinical nurse specialist in the discipline. She was also a phenomenal advisor who knew the questions to ask.

"Well, I haven't really had much of a chance to think about it too much. But the other day, I was thinking about my friends. I was thinking about the freshmen I am a mentor for. They are all a little different than my fellow nursing students and me. I think it has something to do with the things we are exposed to during nursing school."

Dr. Samuelson nodded, silently saying, "Go on."

"As you know," I continued, "we see a lot during nursing school. Heck, nurses in general see a lot. We see dying patients, families that are grieving, families that are in massive arguments, children with terrible illnesses – we see all kinds of emotional things. And at some level, I feel like we grow up a little quicker, at least how we view life. As one of my nursing professors said the other day, we are forced to deal with situations that a lot of people don't deal with until they are in their 30s or 40s, and we are only in our early 20s."

"Interesting perspective," Dr. Samuelson said. "I think you're right in that nursing students are put through an emotional rollercoaster. Not only do you deal with emotion on a daily basis during clinical, but you also have the emotion that goes along with being a student – studying for exams and writing papers. How do you think nursing students can cope with all that they do? What advice would you give an incoming nursing student?"

See, it could never be simple. There were always questions for me. Looking back at all of the conversations I had with Dr. Samuelson, the majority of the time, she was asking me to think deeper and to consider situations or ideas more fully. She was priming me to think critically and also led me to reflect on my life, even without coming out and asking specific questions.

"Well," I began, "for starters, it's absolutely essential for students to share their emotions and experiences with their friends and family, especially their fellow nursing students. And I think it's also important that they keep their advisor in the loop. Knowing that others are feeling the same way helped me a lot," I noted.

She agreed with my response. She knew that I had spent a lot of time in her office sharing my feelings. After my grandfather died, for example, I spent several hours in her office, combing over the details, trying to make sense of what had happened. I couldn't understand how I snapped out of grandson mode and into nurse mode. "How in the world could I have been so removed from the situation?" I had asked. She listened to me and let me "dump" my brain. In just the right places, she added in comments, helping me to process the event. Aside from the experience with my grandfather, I had come to her with many other questions, comments, and concerns, and she always was willing to lend an ear.

I also spent a lot of time talking with my peers. We talked about the sad situations we experienced and supported each other. There were a lot of hugs, and there were tears. But we all felt support because of our "network" of nursing students. We were always just a text or phone call away from each other.

We continued chatting about the previous four years, reflecting on our memories together and also discussing the coming years. About an hour and 15 minutes later, our "meeting" was over. The only reason I had to leave was because another student had arrived for a meeting with Dr. Samuelson.

Before I could get out the door, however, Dr. Samuelson said, "Oh, by the way, I've got a great graduation gift for you, but you'll have to wait until your graduation party," she said with a smile. "It's something only we could appreciate."

"That's appropriate," I commented. "Nobody has ever really understood the two of us, have they?"

She just grinned.

As it turned out, she had been at an antique shop and found a box full of letters written in the 1940s to a nursing student from what seems to be the girl's close friends and family. These letters, which appear to only have cost three cents to mail, were fascinating, revealing what it was like for a nursing students in those days. This was a perfect graduation gift, and in writing this book, I even thought about how that student's letters compare to my stories. As it turns out, many of the struggles and emotions this student in the 1940s experienced, I too experienced during nursing school.

In one letter, for instance, what seems to be one of her close friends who is already a nurse says, "I find most girls think the first year is the hardest, so I do hope you are doing O. K." In another letter, the writer pens, "I do hope you are feeling better. When will you hear about your test? Is this one the only one you were afraid of? Just keep your chin up and be determined that you are going to get what you want."

It seems like nursing tests more than seven decades ago also created fear for students and that emotions ran high. Indeed, this graduation gift was one of the most sentimental. Dr. Samuelson outdid herself, once again.

Ch. 30:
Walking Across the Stage

Graduation was a rather surreal moment. After giving about 120% throughout the previous four years, my days of classes and meetings and nights of care planning and studying were over. It seemed so abrupt and so final.

The Decatur Civic Center was nice and cold. It had to be, as we were all "garbed up" in graduation gowns, and it was quite warm outside. After filing in, we listened to the usual introductions and concentrated on what the speakers had to say. Then, the handing out of diplomas began. (Actually, we were just handed a nice diploma display folder with a letter in it that said we would receive our diploma in a few weeks.) As the students from the School of Music made their way across the stage, I became contemplative.

I had accepted a job already and knew where I would be working after graduation, but still, I distinctly remember asking myself, "What's next?"

Sure, I knew I would begin working in the hospital and would learn a great deal in my new position. But what unexpected events would occur? Where would I *really* be in five years? Would I meet someone that I would soon fall in love with? If I did, would that change my plans of further education? Sure, I had goals, but as I found during my undergraduate years, there is no telling what opportunities will present themselves and how life might change.

When I started nursing school, I had no idea how patients like Jacob and the Mulgrews would affect me. There was no way for me to have known how I would feel when I sat with a patient like Betty Wortzler who was dying. I had no idea that I would feel so empowered by hearing a patient like Dianne Winikie simply say, "thanks." I didn't realize just how trusted nurses really are until I met the family of patients like Mr. Smith and Tyrone Davis, and there was no way I could have predicted I would name a stuffed dog "George." In short, I had no idea how nursing school would impact me and what I would learn. Sure, I thought I had an idea at the beginning, but I really didn't.

This all certainly left me questioning my future. What would it *really* be like when I started working as a "real" nurse? Would my plans change? When would I go back to earn my master's degree? I had an idea, but what if things changed?

The questions continued in my head, but before I knew it, the College of Professional Studies was up, and it was time to walk across the stage.

"Will the candidates for the degree Bachelor of Science in Nursing please rise," I heard. "Chairman Dukeman, I present to you today the following candidates who are eligible for a Bachelor of Science degree in nursing from the College of Professional Studies."

"On behalf of the faculty of Millikin University and as authorized by the board of trustees, I confer upon you the degree Bachelor of Science in nursing with all the rights and privileges pertaining thereto," Chairman Dukeman announced. With that, our line of nursing graduates made our way to the stage.

Just moments later, I heard those words that I will never forget: "Graduating *summa cum laude*, John Robert Blakeman." The time had come. All of my semesters of hard work – all of the friends, professors and patients – it had all been worth it.

As I walked back to my seat, I couldn't help but smile. Sure, I knew I had a lot in front of me, but I also had a lot behind me. I had been through a lot, and I had made it. I felt like I had achieved my goals and even exceeded them in many ways. For this instant, I would relish the moment. Walking across the stage switched my focus from thinking about the future to thinking about the past. When I returned to my seat, I looked around and could see some of my nursing professors sitting in their chairs with all of their regalia on, beaming proudly at all of us. They were just as proud of us as our parents. They knew what we had been through, too, and they knew this day was special.

Later in the day, I met with Ian and Richie, two of my fellow nursing students, and Ian's girlfriend, at one of the local "hole in the wall" taverns that we enjoyed going to just to talk about life and contemplate the problems of the world. It was a quiet place that we had been to many times, and during my time at Millikin, I had met there with some of my friends outside of nursing for the same reasons – to see what was going on in their lives and to hear about their plans for the future. I regarded this establishment as a place to think – like a library – not as a place to drink oneself silly.

Ian and Richie were already there when I arrived. We exchanged the typical pleasantries and talked about our plans for the future.

"Can you believe you guys are done?" Ian's girlfriend asked.

The three of us all sat silently for a few seconds, and then kind of laughed together. "Yes. It's about time it's over," Ian responded. "We've been through enough."

"Yeah. At times it felt like it was never going to end," I added, "But holy cow. It's finally sinking in that it is over."

We had reached an end, sure. But it wasn't *the* end. I think we all knew that we had reached a beginning, too. We had gone to nursing school to learn how to be exceptional nurses – not just nurses that do their required, basic duties and then go home – but nurses that would go the extra two miles for our patients. Our bachelor's education was complete, but now it was time for us to implement all we had learned. Once we passed our licensing exam, we would be working with patients – with *our* patients that we were assigned. We would no longer have one or two patients to care for. Instead, we would be caring for large teams of patients – some of us eight or more patients at a time.

Given all that we had learned, we were ready to make a difference. We knew we *could* make a difference. We knew we *would* make a difference. We *are* making a difference today – one patient at a time.

AFTERWORD

Cardiovascular nursing has always been on the top of my interest list. During pathophysiology and my medical-surgical nursing course, I found the sections discussing the heart and blood vessels the most appealing. The story of landing my first nursing position is fairly short but also fairly awesome. I applied on a Monday, had an interview about a week and a half later, and I accepted the job the following Monday. The job offer actually came on the exact day that my grandpa died. Sometimes I wonder if there was some sort of final message in this occurrence, or if it was just coincidence. Of course, I would like to believe it was a message to me.

The unit that I started my career on was a cardiothoracic-surgical step-down unit and also dealt with patients that had routine cardiac diagnoses like heart failure and atrial fibrillation, a common heart arrhythmia, where the top and bottom part of the heart are not beating correctly and the heart rate can sometimes become too quick. I was lucky to end up on a unit with great support. I was able to work closely with my nurse colleagues, and they helped develop my confidence and further skill as a nurse.

I learned several important lessons.

First, whether or not students enjoy mental health nursing, it is incredibly important. Interpersonal communication is absolutely essential in the clinical setting.

Second, it is very important for nursing students to realize that they, very soon, will be the last line of defense for their patients. In other words, nursing school should be taken very seriously.

Almost every single shift I work, I flash back to memories of nursing school. Whether I'm seeing a unique assessment finding – homonymous hemianopsia, where a patient only sees out of half of their visual fields – or synthesizing laboratory data to help figure out what is "going on" with a patient, nursing school certainly prepared me.

I really like this quotation by Arthur Williams, Jr.
"I'm not telling you it's going to be easy. I'm telling you it's going to be worth it."

That one quotation really sums up nursing. In fact, I have seen several nursing student-related t-shirts and Facebook pages with this quotation.

It's true. Nursing school is not necessarily "fun." It's definitely hard work. At times, emotions can run higher than they have ever run before. But that emotion goes both ways. Sometimes it's great joy and satisfaction; other times, it's sadness and even anger. But in the end, it's worth it.

The patients I have been able to work with and the families I have interacted with have taught me why I really chose nursing. It's a privilege to do what I do, day in and day out. Do I have "those days" where things do not go quite as planned? Do I get stressed out? Have I had patients code on my watch? Oh yes. But I never come home thinking that I did not make a difference. As nurses, and as a member of the health care team in general, no matter where we work, and no matter who we work with, we can always make a positive difference.

So, yes. Those long days and sometimes longer nights were worth it. Those thirty page care plans, lengthy assessment forms and brain-taxing exams were worth it. The tears, venting to my friends, the anger, the stress? Yes. All worth it . . . worth it because today, I am a nurse.

A CONCLUDING THOUGHT

True or False: It is possible to judge whether someone is a "good" nurse by how good he or she is at starting an IV.

For years, I have heard people comment on having a "good" nurse because their nurse was good at starting an IV or inserting a Foley catheter or giving an injection. But does this really solely define a "good" nurse? Should a person jump to requesting a different nurse, simply because his or her nurse is not the best at a task?

As I've grown to understand the art and science of nursing, I've come to realize that nursing is much more than what we see on TV or even what we observe with our eyes in the hospital, and it's what goes on inside a nurse's brain even more than what happens when the nurse is touching a patient that should concern us and ultimately define a "good" nurse.

While it is certainly nice from the patient perspective for a nurse to successfully start an IV the first time, this aspect is only one small fragment of that nurse's ability. I've known nurses that aren't the best at nursing tasks (starting IVs, giving injections, making beds) but that are very good at what I think is one of the hardest aspects for society at large to grasp when it comes to nursing: critical thinking and clinical thinking – utilizing various sources of information to best meet the needs of the patient.

Coming from the perspective of a bachelor's degree (and soon-to-be master's degree) prepared nurse, nursing is much more than what is seen by patients and portrayed in the media. We do not simply learn how to give baths and administer medications (though these, too, are important elements). Bachelor's nursing education generally consists of several science courses, such as chemistry, biochemistry, microbiology, anatomy and physiology and pathophysiology.

We take courses on pharmacology, health assessment, health policy and economics. Further, we learn about evidence-based practice and how to translate research into practice in order to provide the best possible care to patients. We spend semester after semester learning how to therapeutically communicate with patients and think about how to best meet a patient where he or she is coming from. And the list goes on...

Being good at starting an IV does not catch early signs of trouble in a patient. It doesn't prevent a medication error. It doesn't help a nurse spot an adverse reaction to a medication or complication from a surgery. It does not tell the nurse when he or she needs to notify the physician that something is going wrong with a patient. It doesn't help a nurse think proactively. It doesn't help the nurse communicate therapeutically with a patient. This is where "behind-the-scenes" nursing begins, and the majority of it occurs inside the nurse's brain. Many times, nurses collaborate together and with the interdisciplinary health care team (social workers, physical/occupational/speech therapy, case managers, respiratory therapy, physicians, etc.) to reach the best possible solutions, as well.

Please, please believe me; it's not all about tasks. It's about problem solving and recognizing and fitting together pieces of the puzzle, and all of this action occurs, usually, out of sight of the patient. The good nurse is synthesizing vast amounts of "data" (e.g., vital signs, laboratory values, radiology reports, signs/symptoms) to critically analyze the situation and do what is best for the patient. It's also about therapeutic and empathic communication that not only builds trust between the nurse and the patient but that helps the patient heal.

This short note is not meant to suggest that being good at nursing tasks is not important. Truly, I would prefer a nurse that is superb at everything. However, if I had to select a nurse and could only pick between one that was really good at tasks and one that was a phenomenal critical/clinical thinker, I'd choose the latter. This idea can be applied to a whole host of other professionals, too – not just nursing.

So, I implore you. The next time you are in a health care setting as a patient, visitor or staff member (yes, health care workers are guilty of it too), remember that a nurse's ability to do a task well does not define him or her as a nurse. It is only one small piece of the puzzle. Ask the nurse questions. Try to find out what is going on in the nurse's head. Then, you will be able to see the true skill level of the nurse.

REFERENCES

Aiken, L. H., Clarke, S. P., Cheung, R. B., Sloane, D. M., & Silber, J. H. (2003). Educational levels of hospital nurses and surgical patient mortality. *Journal of the American Medical Association, 290*(12), 1617-1623.

American Nurses Association. (2012). The nursing process. Retrieved from: http://nursingworld.org/EspeciallyForYou/What-is-Nursing/Tools-You-Need/Thenursingprocess.html

Bretscheider, J. G. & McCoy, N. L. (1988). Sexual interest and behavior in healthy 80- to 102-year-olds. *Archives of Sexual Behavior, 17,* 109-129.

Institute of Medicine. (2010). *The future of nursing: Leading change, advancing health.* Washington, D. C.: The National Academies Press.

Johns Hopkins. (2011). STDs in baby boomers and beyond. *The Johns Hopkins Medical Letter: Health After 50, 23*(3), 7.

Lenahan, P. M. & Ellwood, A. L. (2004). Sexual health and aging. *Clinics in Family Practice, 6*(4), 917-939.

Morley, J. E. & Tariq, S. H. (2003). Sexuality and disease. *Clinics in Geriatric Medicine, 19*(3), 563-573.

New England Healthcare Institute. (2009). Thinking outside the pillbox: A system-wide approach to improving patient medication adherence for chronic disease. Retrieved from http://www.nehi.net/uploads/full_report/pa_issue_brief__final.pdf

Tortora, G. J. & Derrickson, B. (2009). *Principles of anatomy and physiology* (12th ed.). Hoboken, NJ: John Wiley & Sons.

Wooten-Bielski, K. (1999). HIV and AIDS in older adults. *Geriatric Nursing, 20*(5), 268-272.

RECOMMENDED READING FOR NURSING STUDENTS

Final Gifts: Understanding the Special Awareness, Needs, and Communications of the Dying
By Maggie Callanan and Patricia Kelley

The Immortal Life of Henrietta Lacks
By Rebecca Skloot

The Spirit Catches You and You Fall Down: A Hmong Child, Her American Doctors, and the Collision of Two Cultures
By Anne Fadiman

A Nurse's Story
By Tilda Shalof

Tending Lives: Nurses on the Medical Front
By Echo Heron

From Novice to Expert
By Patricia Benner

Hot Lights, Cold Steel: Life, Death and Sleepless Nights in a Surgeon's First Years
By Michael J. Collins

Something for the Pain: Compassion and Burnout in the ER
By Paul Austin

Appendix:
John's Activities/Courses by
Semester
(number of credit hours in parenthesis)

Fall 2009:

General Chemistry (3) + Lab (1)
Public Speaking (3)
University Seminar (3)
Critical Writing, Reading and Research I (3)
Introductory Psychology (3)
Independent Research

Spring 2010:

Essentials of Organic & Biochemistry (3) + Lab (1)
Intro to the Modern World (3)
Critical Writing, Reading and Research II (3)
Lifespan Development (3)
Social Work Theory and Practice (3)
Basic ECG Rhythm Interpretation (1)
Independent Research

Summer 2010:

Social Issues in Healthcare (3)

Fall 2010:

Human Anatomy & Physiology (4) + Lab (0)
Principles of Microbiology (4) + Lab (0)
Principles of Psychopathology (3)
Practice with Diverse Populations (3)
Independent Study Nursing (2)
Curriculum Committee
Independent Research

Winter 2010:
>*Social Gerontology (3)*

Spring 2011:
>*Intro Practicum in Nursing (5) + Clinical*
>*Human Anatomy & Physiology II (4) + Lab (0)*
>*Health Assessment (3)*
>*Intro to Sociology (3)*
>*Curriculum Committee*
>*Independent Research*

Fall 2011:
>*Mental Health Nursing (9) + Clinical*
>*Pathophysiologic Concepts for Nurses (3)*
>*Elementary Probability and Statistics (3)*
>*Intro to Visual Culture (3)*
>*Student Welfare Committee*
>*Student Senate – Senator, College of Professional Studies*
>*Independent Research*

Spring 2012:
>*Parent-Child Nursing (9) + Clinical*
>*Pharmacology (3)*
>*Global Approaches to Medicine & Healthcare (3)*
>*Biostatistical Methods (3) [graduate course]*
>*Student Welfare Committee*
>*Student Senate – Senator, College of Professional Studies*
>*Independent Research*

Summer 2012:
>*Summer Nursing Experience (2)*

Fall 2012:

Medical-Surgical Nursing (9) + Clinical
Issues: Nursing Research & Management (4)
Nursing & Interdisciplinary Theory (3) [graduate course]
Curriculum Committee
Student Senate – Vice President of Academic Affairs
Independent Research

Spring 2013:

Community Health Nursing (9) + Clinical
Transition to Professional Nursing (1)
Intercultural Communication (3)
Principles of Teaching & Learning (3) [graduate course]
Curriculum Committee
Student Senate – Vice President of Academic Affairs
Independent Research

ABOUT THE AUTHOR

John R. Blakeman is a registered professional nurse, practicing in Illinois. He currently works on a cardiothoracic-surgical step-down and general cardiology unit. He is a graduate student at Millikin University in Decatur, Illinois, earning a Master of Science in Nursing (MSN) degree in the nurse educator track, with an anticipated graduation of fall 2015. Additionally, he serves as a graduate assistant for the Millikin School of Nursing.

John's MSN project is focused on the symptoms women experience in the weeks and months prior to myocardial infarction ("heart attack"). He has also spent time researching bedside electrocardiogdraphic monitoring, effective hand hygiene programs, and evidence-based practice implementation methods.

He earned his Bachelor of Science in Nursing from Millikin University, graduating *summa cum laude*. During his undergraduate tenure at Millikin, John enjoyed a scholar's career, receiving several awards, including the Dr. J. Roger Miller Leadership Award and the Scovill Prize. Additionally, he has published an academic journal article in the *Journal of Psychosocial Nursing and Mental Health Services*, as well as a letter to the editor in the *Journal of Nursing Education*.

In his spare time, he enjoys reading, writing, socializing with friends and family, listening to music from diverse genres, and exploring nature.

Made in the USA
Lexington, KY
28 February 2015